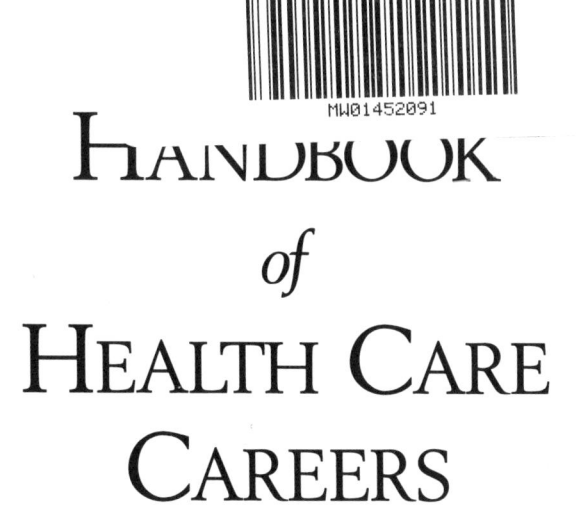

Handbook
of
Health Care Careers

VGM's HANDBOOK *of* HEALTH CARE CAREERS

edited by Annette Selden

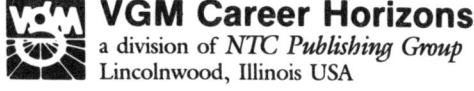

VGM Career Horizons
a division of *NTC Publishing Group*
Lincolnwood, Illinois USA

Library of Congress Cataloging-in-Publication Data

VGM's handbook of health care careers / edited by Annette Selden.
    p.   cm.
    ISBN 0-8442-4148-2
    1. Medicine—Vocational guidance. 2. Medical personnel—Vocational guidance. I. Selden, Annette. II. VGM Career Horizons. III. Title: Handbook of health care careers.
    [DNLM: 1. Career Choice—handbooks. 2. Health Occupations—handbooks. W 39 V597]
R690.V45   1992
610'.23—dc20
DNLM/DLC   92-49633
for Library of Congress   CIP

Published by VGM Career Horizons, a division of NTC Publishing Group.
© 1993 by NTC Publishing Group, 4255 West Touhy Avenue,
Lincolnwood (Chicago), Illinois 60646-1975 U.S.A.
All rights reserved. No part of this book may be reproduced, stored
in a retrieval system, or transmitted in any form or by any means,
electronic, mechanical, photocopying, recording or otherwise, without
the prior permission of NTC Publishing Group.
manufactured in the United States of America.

2 3 4 5 6 7 8 9 0 VP 9 8 7 6 5 4 3 2 1

Foreword

It is difficult to think of a more demanding career than health care. Professional medical personnel are held to a high standard of excellence. They are expected to master their specialization and deliver high-tech medical care without ever forgetting the human element of their jobs.

Yet, for those who are willing to devote the requisite time and energy, health care can be an excellent career choice. Demand for health care professionals is increasing in most fields, offering practitioners good job security and improved salaries and benefits.

Health care also offers a less tangible benefit: the opportunity to engage in exceptionally rewarding and meaningful work.

Good luck to you in your search for the right health care career.

The Editors of VGM

Contents

How to Use This Book	ix
Biomedical Engineer	1
Chiropractor	3
Cytotechnologist	5
Dental Assistant	7
Dental Hygienist	9
Dental Laboratory Technician	11
Dentist	13
Dietician	15
Electrocardiograph (EKG) Technician	17
Electroencephalograph (EEG) Technologist	19
Emergency Medical Technician	21
Health Services Manager	23
Medical Assistant	26
Medical Laboratory Technologist	28
Medical Record Technician	31
Medical Secretary	33
Nuclear Medicine Technologist	34
Nurse, Licensed Practical	37
Nurse, Registered	38
Nursing Aide	41
Occupational Therapist	42
Ophthalmic Laboratory Technician	45
Ophthalmologist	46
Optician, Dispensing	48
Optometrist	50
Osteopathic Physician	52
Pharmacist	54
Pharmacologist	56

Contents

Physical Therapist	58
Physician	60
Physician Assistant	62
Podiatrist	64
Prosthetist and Orthotist	66
Psychiatrist	68
Psychologist	70
Radiologic (X-Ray) Technologist	73
Recreational Therapist	75
Rehabilitation Counselor	77
Respiratory Therapist	79
Speech Pathologist and Audiologist	82
Surgical Technologist	83
Veterinarian	85
Appendix: Resumes, Application Forms, Cover Letters, and Interviews	89

How to Use This Book

VGM's Handbook of Health Care Careers contains vital information on popular careers in health care. Each career has been carefully researched and described in text that is easy to understand. The careers are listed in alphabetical order for easy reference, and each is described in the following fashion:

- ◇ *The Job.* A general description of what the job is like and what persons in the field are expected to do.
- ◇ *Places of Employment and Working Conditions.* Where major employers in the field are located and what type of work environment to expect, i.e. office work, outdoor work, urban location, rural location. Typical working hours are also given.
- ◇ *Qualifications, Education, and Training.* How to qualify for a job in the field, what type of education is necessary, and any special training that may help you get a start in the field.
- ◇ *Potential and Advancement.* The approximate number of persons employed in the field nationwide, projections on whether the field will grow or shrink in the upcoming years, and typical paths of advancement for workers.
- ◇ *Income.* The most current salary figures available, for beginners in the field and for experienced workers. Keep in mind that such figures are subject to change, due primarily to supply and demand within the labor force and to inflation. Be sure to check with various employers and associations for the most recent figures while conducting your job search.
- ◇ *Additional Sources of Information.* Names and addresses of associations and other groups that can supply more information about careers in the field. These organizations can be very helpful, so be sure to contact them if you need additional information.

This handy reference book allows you to compare and contrast various careers in health care all within one volume. You can use it to find out about fields that may already interest you, or you can read it cover to cover in order to explore a variety of career paths that you might find appealing.

The appendix in the back of the book helps you with resumes, application forms, cover letters, and interviews. Once you have settled on a particular career path, be sure to use this information to prepare yourself to go after a job.

Biomedical Engineer

The Job Biomedical engineers apply engineering principles to medical and health-related problems.

Most engineers in this field are involved in research. They work with life scientists, chemists, and members of the medical profession to design and develop medical devices such as artificial hearts, pacemakers, dialysis machines, and lasers for surgery. Others work for private industry in the development, design, and sale of medical instruments and devices.

Biomedical engineers with computer expertise adapt computers to medical needs and design and build systems to modernize laboratory and clinical procedures. Some work for the National Aeronautics and Space Administration developing life support and medical monitoring systems for astronauts.

Places of Employment and Working Conditions Some phases of this work may be unpleasant when working with certain illnesses or medical conditions.

Qualifications, Education, and Training The ability to think analytically, a capacity for details, and the ability to work as part of a team are all necessary. Good communication skills are important.

Mathematics and the sciences must be emphasized in high school. A bachelor's degree in engineering is the minimum requirement in this field. In a typical curriculum, the first two years are spent in the study of basic sciences such as physics and chemistry and mathematics, introductory engineering, and some liberal arts courses. The remaining years are usually devoted to specialized engineering courses. For this field that means a sound background in mechanical, electrical, industrial, or chemical engineering plus additional specialized biomedical training.

Engineering programs can last from four to six years. Those that require five or six years to complete may award a master's degree or may provide a cooperative plan of study plus practical work experience with a nearby industry.

All states require licensing of engineers whose work may affect life, health, or property or who offer their services to the public. Those who are licensed, about one-third of all engineers, are called registered engineers. Requirements for licensing include graduation from an accredited engineering school, four years of experience, and an examination.

Biomedical Engineer

Potential and Advancement There are only about 4,000 biomedical engineers. Substantial growth is expected, but, since the field is relatively small, few actual job openings will occur. Those with advanced degrees will have the best job opportunities.

Income Starting salaries in private industry average $25,000 a year with a master's degree and $32,000 or more with a Ph.D.

Additional Sources of Information

Accreditation Board for Engineering and Technology
345 East 47th Street
New York, NY 10017

Alliance for Engineering in Medicine and Biology
1101 Connecticut Avenue, NW
Suite 700
Washington, DC 20036

American Society for Engineering Education
11 Dupont Circle, NW
Suite 200
Washington, DC 20036

Biomedical Engineering Society
P.O. Box 2399
Culver City, CA 90230

Junior Engineering and Technical Society (JETS)
1420 King Street
Suite 405
Alexandria, VA 22314

National Society of Professional Engineers
1420 King Street
Alexandria, VA 22314

Society of Women Engineers
345 East 47th Street
Room 305
New York, NY 10017

Chiropractor

The Job Chiropractors treat patients by manual manipulations (called adjustments) of parts of the body, especially the spinal column. This system of treatment is based on the theory that pressure on nerves that pass from the spinal cord to different parts of the body interferes with nerve impulses and their functioning, causing disorders in parts of the body. By means of certain manipulations of the vertebrae, the chiropractor seeks to relieve the pressure on specific nerves and thus remove the cause of a specific ailment.

Most chiropractors also employ x-rays to aid in locating the source of an ailment. They use supplementary treatment with water, light, or heat therapy and may prescribe diet, exercise, and rest. Drugs and surgery are not used in this system of treatment.

Newly licensed chiropractors often start their careers by working in salaried positions—as assistants to established practitioners or in chiropractic clinics.

Since a chiropractic practice can be conducted on a part-time basis, it is a good field for people with family responsibilities.

Places of Employment and Working Conditions Chiropractors often locate in small communities, with about half of all chiropractors practicing in cities of 50,000 or less. California, Oregon, Colorado, Wyoming, Arizona, and New Mexico have the most chiropractors.

Most chiropractors are in private practice, which allows them to schedule their own working hours. Evening and weekend hours are sometimes necessary to accommodate their patients.

Qualifications, Education, and Training Manual dexterity rather than strength is necessary for a chiropractor. A keen sense of observation, an ability to deal with people, and a sympathetic manner with the sick are also important.

High school courses in science are important, and the two years of college required before entrance into chiropractic school must include chemistry, biology, and physics.

There are 14 chiropractic colleges that are accredited by the Council on Chiropractic Education; three others are working toward accreditation. The four-year course of study emphasizes courses in manipulation and spinal ad-

Chiropractor

justment, but most schools also offer a broad curriculum that includes basic and clinical sciences.

The first two years of study include classroom and laboratory work in anatomy, physiology, and biochemistry. The last two years are devoted to practical experience in college clinics. The degree of D.C. (doctor of chiropractic) is awarded upon completion of the course.

All chiropractors must be licensed to practice. In addition to a state board examination, licensing requirements usually include two years of college and the successful completion of an accredited four-year chiropractic course, as described above. Some states also require a basic science examination.

Potential and Advancement There are about 36,000 practicing chiropractors. This number will increase because the profession is gaining greater public acceptance. Enrollment in chiropractic colleges has increased in recent years. New chiropractors may find it increasingly difficult to establish a practice in areas where other practitioners are located; the best opportunities will be in areas with few established chiropractors.

Income As in any type of independent practice, earnings are relatively low in the beginning. Experienced chiropractors earn about $64,000 a year, with many earning considerably more.

Additional Sources of Information

American Chiropractic Association
1701 Clarendon Boulevard
Arlington, VA 22209

Council on Chiropractic Education
4401 Westown Parkway
Suite 120
West Des Moines, IA 50265

Cytotechnologist

The Job Cytotechnologists are specialized medical technologists who assist physicians by performing laboratory tests to determine body cell abnormalities. An abnormality in a body cell may indicate cancer, and the cytotechnologist's detection of a malignancy may mean the difference between life and death for a patient.

After receiving a physician's order for laboratory tests, the cytotechnologist prepares slides of body cells and microscopically examines them to determine whether there are any cell abnormalities. He or she then interprets the results of the tests and sends them back to the physician. The physician uses the test results to inform the patient of the absence or presence of a disease and to decide what course of treatment will be most effective.

Most cytotechnologists work in hospitals, but others work in independent laboratories, physicians' offices, clinics, health maintenance organizations (HMOs), public health agencies, pharmaceutical firms, and research institutions.

Places of Employment and Working Conditions
Cytotechnologists are in demand in all areas of the country, with the largest concentrations of jobs in metropolitan areas.

Cytotechnologists work in clean, well-lighted laboratories. Sometimes they must work with infectious specimens that have to be handled with great care. Odors are sometimes present in the laboratory, and workers must cope with the stress of performing their job both quickly and accurately.

Cytotechnologists who work in hospitals or laboratories that operate 24 hours a day may have to work day, evening, or night shifts. Weekend and holiday work is usually required since laboratories operate 365 days a year.

Qualifications, Education, and Training
Cytotechnologists must be accurate and dependable and must have the ability to form judgments based on the tests they perform and cope with pressure. They must be detail oriented and have problem-solving capabilities. Good interpersonal communication skills are also important.

A bachelor's degree with a major in medical technology or the life sciences and specialized training in cytotechnology is necessary for entry-level jobs. This educational training is offered in colleges, universities, and hospitals. Those who are interested in this career field should make sure that the program they are taking is accredited by the Committee on Allied Health Education and Accreditation (CAHEA) in cooperation with the National Accrediting Agency for

Clinical Laboratory Sciences (NAACLS). They also should be aware that some states require workers to be licensed or registered.

Potential and Advancement   The field of cytotechnology offers excellent job prospects. There is currently a shortage of workers in this field, and the number of cytotechnology students is on the decline. Cytotechnologists are in demand, and the supply is currently not sufficient.

With graduate education, cytotechnologists may advance in several ways. They may be promoted to supervisory positions in large hospitals and laboratories. Other workers move on to employment with manufacturers of home diagnostic testing kits and laboratory equipment and supplies.

Income   Starting salaries for cytotechnologists average about $20,000 a year. Experienced cytotechnologists earn an average of about $26,000 annually.

Additional Sources of Information

American Society for Medical Technology
2021 L Street, NW
Washington, DC 20036

American Medical Technologists
710 Higgins Road
Park Ridge, IL 60068

American Society of Cytology
1015 Chestnut Street
Suite 1518
Philadelphia, PA 19107

Committee on Allied Health and Accreditation
535 North Dearborn Street
Chicago, IL 60610

Dental Assistant

The Job   Dental assistants work with dentists and oral hygienists as they examine and treat patients. They are usually employed in private dental offices and often combine office duties, such as making appointments, maintaining patient records, and billing, with chairside assisting.

Dental assistants prepare instruments and materials for treatment procedures, process dental x-ray films, sterilize instruments, prepare plaster casts of teeth from impressions taken by the dentists, and sometimes provide oral medications to teeth and gums, remove excess filling materials from surfaces of teeth, and fit rubber isolation dams on individual teeth before treatment by the dentist.

Dental assistants are also employed in dental schools, hospital dental departments, state and local public health departments, and private clinics. The federal government employs them in the Public Health Service, the Veterans Administration, and the armed forces.

Most dental assistants are women. Opportunities for part-time work are numerous, making this a good field for people with family responsibilities.

Places of Employment and Working Conditions   Dental assistants are employed in communities of all sizes with the most job opportunities in large metropolitan areas.

A 40-hour workweek is usual for full-time dental assistants, but this includes some evening and Saturday hours in most dental offices.

Qualifications, Education, and Training   Neatness and the ability to help people relax are important personal qualities.

High school courses in biology, chemistry, health, typing, and office practices are helpful.

Most dental assistants acquire their skills on the job. Office skills often provide entry into a dental office where a beginner handles appointments, acts as receptionist, and performs routine clerical and recordkeeping chores. Dental assisting skills are then acquired over a period of time.

An increasing number of dental assistants are acquiring their training in formal programs at junior and community colleges and vocational and technical schools. Most of these programs require one year or less to complete. Two-year programs include some liberal arts courses and offer an associate's degree upon

7

Dental Assistant

completion. Some private schools offer four- to six-month courses in dental assisting, but these are not accredited by the Commission on Dental Accreditation. Dental assistants who receive their training in the armed forces usually qualify for civilian jobs.

Graduates of accredited programs may receive professional recognition by completing an examination given by the Dental Assisting National Board. They are then designated as certified dental assistants.

Potential and Advancement There are about 166,000 people working as dental assistants; one-third work part-time. Job opportunities should be excellent for the future, especially for graduates of formal training programs.

Dental assistants in large dental offices or clinics are sometimes promoted to supervisory positions. Some advance by fulfilling the educational requirements necessary to become dental hygienists. Others teach in or administer dental assisting education programs.

Income Salaries vary widely from community to community and depend on training and experience, job responsibilities and duties, and size of dental practice.

The average income for full-time dental assistants is about $267 a week.

Additional Sources of Information

American Dental Assistants Association
919 North Michigan Avenue
Suite 3400
Chicago, IL 60611

Dental Assisting National Board, Inc.
216 East Ontario Street
Chicago, IL 60611

Dental Hygienist

The Job Dental hygienists are involved in both clinical dental work and education with specific responsibilities governed by the state in which the hygienist is employed.

Working as part of a dental health team under the supervision of a dentist, a dental hygienist may clean and polish a patient's teeth, removing deposits and stains at the same time; apply medication for the prevention of tooth decay; take and develop x-rays; make model impressions of teeth for study; take medical and dental histories; and provide instruction for patient self-care, diet, and nutrition. In some states, pain control and restorative procedures may also be performed by dental hygienists.

Some dental hygienists work in school systems where they examine students' teeth, assist dentists in determining necessary dental treatment, and report their findings to parents. They give instruction in proper mouth care and develop classroom or assembly programs on oral health.

Most dental hygienists are employed in private dental offices; many are employed part-time.

Other employers are public health agencies, industrial plants, clinics and hospitals, dental hygienist schools, the federal government, and the armed forces (those with a bachelor's degree are commissioned officers). A few dental hygienists are involved in research projects.

Places of Employment and Working Conditions Dental hygienists work in communities of all sizes.

They usually work a 35- to 40-hour week; those employed by a dentist in private practice usually have some weekend and evening hours. Dental hygienists are required to stand for a good part of the working day.

Certain health protection procedures are important for anyone working in this field. These include regular medical checkups and strict adherence to established procedures for disinfection and use of x-ray equipment.

Qualifications, Education, and Training An enjoyment of people and the ability to put a patient at ease are strong assets. Manual dexterity is necessary. Good health, personal cleanliness and neatness, and stamina are very important.

High school courses recommended for anyone interested in a career in this field include biology, chemistry, health, and mathematics.

Requirements for admission to dental hygienist schools vary. Some hygienist schools that offer a bachelor's degree require one or two prior years of college.

Dental Hygienist

There are 197 programs in dental hygiene in the United States that are accredited by the Commission on Dental Accreditation. Students in dental hygienist programs study anatomy, physiology, chemistry, pharmacology, nutrition, tissue structure, gum diseases, dental materials, and clinical dental hygiene. Liberal arts courses are also part of the program. Most programs grant an associate's degree with some schools awarding a bachelor's degree. Several schools offer master's degree programs in dental hygiene or related fields.

Licensing is required for all dental hygienists; all states require graduation from an accredited dental hygienist school as well as written and clinical examination. To pass the clinical examination, the applicant for licensing is tested on proficiency in performing dental hygiene procedures. Most states will accept a passing grade on the written examination given by the American Dental Association Joint Commission on National Dental Examinations as part of the licensing requirement.

Potential and Advancement

About 91,000 persons work as dental hygienists.

This is a field where current job openings outnumber qualified graduates, and the employment outlook for potential dental hygienists is excellent. An expanding population, increased participation in dental insurance plans, more group practice by dentists, and dental care programs for children will also contribute to a still greater demand for trained dental hygienists in the future. There will also be many opportunities for dental hygienists who desire part-time work and for those willing to work in rural areas.

Income

Dental hygienists working in private dental offices are paid on an hourly, daily, salary, or commission basis.

According to the American Dental Hygienists' Association, half of all hygienists earn between $15,000 and $25,000 a year. Their average hourly pay is $14.61.

Additional Sources of Information

Division of Dentistry
Public Health Service
U.S. Department of Health and Human Services
9000 Rockville Pike
Bethesda, MD 20014

Division of Professional Development
American Dental Hygienists' Association
444 North Michigan Avenue
Suite 3400
Chicago, IL 60611

Dental Laboratory Technician

The Job Dental laboratory technicians are skilled craftsworkers who make dental prosthetics such as crowns, bridges, and dentures according to the specifications of dentists. Some specialized technicians make appliances for straightening teeth and treating speech impediments while others make and repair contoured metal frames and retainers for teeth used in removable partial dentures.

Dentists send their requests along with specifications for the item to be made and a mold of the patient's mouth. The technician pours plaster into the mold and lets it set, creating a model of the patient's mouth. After careful examinations and observations of the model, the technician makes a wax tooth or teeth. This wax model is used to cast the metal base of the prosthetic device.

After the cast is poured and the metal base is made, the technician applies porcelain in layers to duplicate the exact color and shape of the tooth. The porcelain is baked on in a kiln. Then the prosthesis is glazed to give it a lacquered finish. The goal of the technician is to recreate exactly the lost tooth or teeth.

In some laboratories, technicians are responsible for completing specific steps in this process while in others, technicians may be responsible for many steps.

Places of Employment and Working Conditions Most dental laboratory technicians work in commercial dental laboratories which are small, privately owned businesses employing fewer than five workers. There are a few larger laboratories employing over 50 workers. Other technicians work in dentists' offices and hospitals that provide dental services.

Work areas are usually clean and well lighted. Although this is generally not a strenuous job, there may be some pressure to meet deadlines. Workweeks are usually 40 hours.

Qualifications, Education, and Training Dental laboratory technicians must be very precise and detail oriented. They must have good vi-

Dental Laboratory Technician

sion and a high degree of manual dexterity. The ability to follow directions is important.

Most dental laboratory technicians learn this craft on the job by performing more basic tasks and progressing to more complicated tasks. It usually takes three to four years to be fully trained.

There are formal programs that offer training in community and junior colleges, vocational-technical institutes, trade schools, high school vocational education programs, apprenticeships, and the armed forces. While the length of these programs and the extent of training vary, it typically takes two years to complete an accredited program. Usually an associate's degree or certificate or diploma are granted upon completion.

There are nearly 60 programs in dental laboratory technology accredited by the Commission on Dental Accreditation in conjunction with the American Dental Association.

Potential and Advancement There are about 51,000 persons working as dental laboratory technicians.

This field will have a slower-than-average growth rate during the next decade. The large growth of the aging population will create some jobs for technicians, but a growing awareness of preventive dental health care and fluoridation of drinking water will result in greater dental health and reduce the need for dental prosthetic devices.

Successful technicians may advance by establishing their own laboratories.

Income Dental laboratory technicians working full-time earn between $15,000 and $25,000 a year. Education, experience, and specialized skills usually bring higher pay.

Additional Sources of Information

Commission on Dental Accreditation
American Dental Association
211 East Chicago Avenue
Chicago, IL 60611

National Association of Dental Laboratories
3801 Mt. Vernon Avenue
Alexandria, VA 22305

Dentist

The Job   Graduates of approved dental schools are entitled to use the designations D.D.S. (doctor of dental surgery) or D.M.D. (doctor of dental medicine).

Most dentists are general practitioners who provide many types of dental care. They examine teeth and mouth tissues to diagnose and treat any diseases or abnormalities of the teeth, gums, supporting bones, and surrounding tissues. They extract teeth, fill cavities, design and insert dentures and inlays, and perform surgery. The dentist, or someone on his or her staff, takes dental and medical histories, cleans teeth, and provides instructions on proper diet and cleanliness to preserve dental health.

About 20 percent of all dentists are specialists. The two largest fields are made up of *orthodontists,* who straighten teeth, and *oral surgeons,* who operate on the mouth and jaws. Other specialties are pediatric dentistry (dentistry for children), periodontics (treatment of the gums), prosthodontics (artificial teeth and dentures), endodontics (root canal therapy), oral pathology (diseases of the mouth), and public health dentistry.

Close to 2,000 civilian dentists are employed by the federal government. These dentists work in hospitals and clinics of the Veterans Administration or in the U.S. Public Health Service.

Places of Employment and Working Conditions   Almost 90 percent of dentists work in private practice, which includes a wide variety of work settings and payment systems. Of the dentists who work outside private practice, half are researchers, teachers, or administrators in dental schools. Others work in hospitals and clinics. The federal government employs about 2,000 dentists, primarily in the hospitals and clinics of the Department of Veterans Affairs and the U.S. Public Health Service.

Qualifications, Education, and Training   Students interested in dentistry as a career should possess a high degree of manual dexterity and scientific ability and have good visual memory and excellent judgment of space and shape.

High school courses should include biology, chemistry, health, and mathematics.

Dental education is very expensive because of the length of time required to earn a dental degree. From three to four years of predental college work in the sciences and humanities is required by dental schools with most successful applicants having a bachelor's or a master's degree. Since competition for admission is stiff, dental schools give considerable weight to the amount of predental education and to college grades. Schools also require personal interviews and recommendations as well as completion of the admission testing program used by all dental schools. In addition, state-supported dental schools usually give preference to residents of the state.

Dental school training lasts four academic years after college or, in some dental colleges, three calendar years. The first two years consist of classroom instruction and laboratory work in anatomy, microbiology, biochemistry, physiology, clinical sciences, and preclinical technique. The remainder of the training period is spent in actual treatment of patients.

A license to practice is required by all states and the District of Columbia. Requirements include a degree from a dental school approved by the Commission on Dental Accreditation and written and practical examinations. A passing grade on the written examination given by the National Board of Dental Examiners is accepted by most states as fulfilling part of the licensing requirements; 20 states will grant a license without examination to dentists already licensed by another state.

In 15 states, dentists who wish to specialize must have two or three years of graduate training, and, in some cases, pass an additional state examination. In the remaining states, a licensed dentist may engage in general or specialized dentistry. In these states, the additional education is also necessary to specialize; however, specialists are regulated by the state dental profession rather than by state licensing.

Potential and Advancement   There are about 142,000 active dentists, 90 percent of them in private practice. The demand for dentists is expected to grow because of population growth, increased awareness of the necessity of dental health, and the expansion of prepaid dental insurance benefits to employees in many industries.

Income   Dentists setting up a new practice can look forward to a few lean years in the beginning. As the practice grows, income will rise rapidly with average yearly earnings around $70,000.

A practice can usually be developed most quickly in small towns where there is less competition from established dentists. Over the long run, however, earnings of dentists in urban areas are higher than earnings in small towns. Specialists generally earn much more than general practitioners, whatever the location, averaging about $100,000 a year.

Additional Sources of Information

American Association of Dental Schools
1625 Massachusetts Avenue, NW
Washington, DC 20036

American Dental Association
Council on Dental Education
211 East Chicago Avenue
Chicago, IL 60611

Division of Dentistry
Public Health Service
U.S. Department of Health and Human Services
9000 Rockville Pike
Bethesda, MD 20014

Dietician

The Job Dieticians plan nutritious and appetizing meals, supervise the preparation and service of food, and manage the purchasing and accounting for their department. Others are involved in research and education.

More than half of all dieticians are employed in hospitals, nursing homes, and other health care facilities. Colleges, universities, school systems, restaurants and cafeterias, large companies that provide food service for their employees, and food processors and manufacturers also employ dieticians.

Some serve as commissioned officers in the armed forces. The federal government also employs dieticians in Veterans Administration hospitals and in the U.S. Public Health Service.

Clinical dieticians form the largest group of dieticians. They plan the diets and supervise the service of meals to meet the various nutritional needs of patients in hospitals, nursing homes, and clinics. They confer with doctors and instruct patients and their families on diet requirements and food preparation.

Management dieticians are responsible for large-scale meal planning and preparation. They purchase food, equipment, and supplies; enforce safety and sanitary regulations; and train and direct food service and supervisory workers. If they are directors of a dietetic department, they may also have budgeting responsibilities, coordinate dietetic service activities with other departments, and set department policy. In a small institution, the duties of administrative and clinical dieticians are usually combined into one position.

Research dieticians evaluate the dietary requirements of specific groups such as the elderly, space travelers, or those with a chronic disease. They also do research in food management and service systems and equipment. *Dietetic educators* teach in medical, dental, and nursing schools.

Nutritionists provide counseling in proper nutrition practices. They work in food industries, educational and health facilities, agricultural agencies, welfare agencies, and community health programs.

Places of Employment and Working Conditions

Dieticians are employed throughout the country with most job opportunities in large metropolitan areas and in areas with large colleges and universities.

Most dieticians work a 40-hour week, but this usually includes some weekend hours. There are many part-time opportunities for dieticians.

Qualifications, Education, and Training

Anyone interested in this career field should have scientific aptitude, organizational and administrative ability, and the ability to work well with people.

High school courses should include biology, chemistry, home economics, mathematics, and some business courses, if possible.

A bachelor's degree in the home economics department with a major in foods and nutrition or institutional management is the basic requirement for a dietician. Almost 260 schools offer undergraduate programs in the field.

A 9- to 12-month internship or a preprofessional practice program should also be completed by any dietician who wants professional recognition. These programs consist primarily of clinical experience under the direction of a qualified dietician. Some colleges and universities have coordinated undergraduate programs that enable students to complete both the clinical and bachelor's degree requirements in four years.

Vocational and technical schools as well as junior colleges also offer training in dietetic services. Students who complete these training courses can work as dietetic assistants or technicians and usually find ample job opportunities.

The American Dietetic Association registers dieticians who meet their established qualifications. The designation RD (registered dietician) is an acknowledgment of a dietician's competence and professional status.

Potential and Advancement

About 40,000 people work as dieticians. Job opportunities, both full- and part-time, should be plentiful through the year 2000.

Dieticians usually advance by moving to larger institutions. In a large institution, they may advance to director of the dietetic department. Some advance by entering some area of clinical specialization. Others become consultants or opt for careers in business and management. Advancement in research and teaching positions usually requires a graduate degree.

Income   Beginners in this field earn about $21,800 a year. Experienced dieticians earn about $29,500 a year.

Additional Source of Information

The American Dietetic Association
216 West Jackson Boulevard
Suite 800
Chicago, IL 60606-6995

Electrocardiograph (EKG) Technician

The Job   By using a machine called an electrocardiograph, EKG technicians record tracings of heartbeats that show the electrical impulses given off by the heart muscle during and between heartbeats. This test is ordered by doctors to determine whether a patient has heart disease; to check the effectiveness of drugs used in treatment; and to study the changes in a patient's heart over a period of time.

The EKG technician attaches electrodes to a patient's chest, arms, and legs and applies a gel between the electrode and the patient's skin so the electrical impulses can be recorded. A stylus or inkpen records the heart's electrical impulses on graph paper as the technician operates different switches on the electrocardiograph and positions electrodes across the patient's chest.

After the technician has performed the test, he or she must prepare it for the physician's use. Technicians working with the most advanced EKG equipment must enter information into a computer for an analysis of the tracing. They must

Electrocardiograph (EKG) Technician

be able to detect errors in the tracings and provide the physician with an accurate reading. They must also point out any abnormalities in the tracings to the physician.

More experienced technicians may perform specialized tests, such as ambulatory monitoring, in which the patient wears a portable EKG while performing normal activities for a period of 24 to 48 hours, or stress testing, in which the patient is tested while walking on a treadmill.

Places of Employment and Working Conditions
EKG technicians work in physicians' offices, cardiac rehabilitation centers, HMOs, and clinics; most work in hospital cardiology departments. While they are employed throughout the country, most job opportunities are in large metropolitan areas.

EKG technicians usually work a 40-hour week, which may include weekend and holiday hours. Those working in hospitals may work evening hours. They spend a great deal of time walking and standing.

Qualifications, Education, and Training
EKG technicians must feel comfortable working with both machines and people. They must be able to follow instructions and cope well in an emergency situation.

EKG technicians must have a high school diploma. Courses in health, biology, and typing will help them in this occupation.

Most EKG technicians receive on-the-job training from an EKG supervisor or cardiologist. Training to perform a basic resting EKG takes four to six weeks. After four to five months, technicians have been trained to administer tests to critically ill patients, interpret graphs, and write reports for physicians. Four more months of training are necessary in order to perform more complicated tests.

Potential and Advancement
Currently, there are about 18,000 EKG technicians, and the field is expected to grow slowly through the year 2000. Improved technology and computerization have increased productivity and decreased demand. Also, many hospitals are cutting back on personnel by training other staff members to perform EKG testing.

Technicians may advance by gaining experience and becoming supervisors, administrators, or managers. Others may transfer to jobs in equipment sales and marketing.

Income
EKG technicians in hospitals, medical schools, and medical centers earn average starting salaries of about $13,044 a year. Those who are more experienced and perform more complicated tests earn more than those who

perform basic ones. Some technicians with more experience earn as much as $24,252 a year.

Additional Source of Information

National Society of Cardiovascular Technology/National Society of Pulmonary Technology (NSCT/NSPT)
1133 15th Street, NW
Suite 1000
Washington, DC 20005

Electroencephalograph (EEG) Technologist

The Job EEG technologists operate an important medical diagnostic machine, the electroencephalograph. Electroencephalographs measure the electrical activity of the human brain, and encephalograms (EEGs), the records produced, are used for several different reasons. Neurologists use them to determine the extent of brain injuries, the effects of infectious brain diseases, and whether the cause of a patient's mental or behavioral problems is organic. Surgeons use EEGs to monitor a patient's condition during surgery, and EEGs are also used to determine whether a patient is clinically dead. Physicians are able to give a better prognosis of a comatose patient's chances for recovery after analyzing an EEG.

EEGs are performed either while patients are resting or ambulatory. Technologists take a medical history from patients and then attach electrodes to their head and body. After making sure that the equipment is working properly, technologists select the correct instrument controls and electrodes that will produce the type of record the physician has ordered. They must be aware of any readings that come from somewhere other than the brain, such as eye movement or interference from other electrical sources, and correct them. They then analyze the test and select sections for the physician to examine. They must know the difference between normal and abnormal brain waves.

Sometimes EEG technologists have supervisory or administrative responsibilities. They also may have to perform EKGs or other procedures.

Electroencephalograph (EEG) Technologist

Places of Employment and Working Conditions Most EEG technologists work in hospitals, but some work in neurology laboratories, neurologists' and neurosurgeons' offices, group medical practices, HMOs, urgent care centers and clinics, and psychiatric facilities.

EEG technologists work in a clean, well-lighted atmosphere. The job can be physically demanding; they spend a great deal of time on their feet and are required to do a lot of bending in working with very ill patients.

Technologists usually have a 5-day, 40-hour workweek with some overtime, but some may have to be on call during evening, weekend, and holiday hours.

Qualifications, Education, and Training EEG technologists must have an aptitude for working with both humans and machinery. They should have manual dexterity, good vision, and writing skills. They must be able to follow directions.

Technologists usually receive their training on the job; a high school diploma is necessary. Some hospitals, medical centers, community colleges, and vocational-technical schools offer one- or two-year formal training programs. Fifteen programs have been accredited by the Joint Review Committee for the Accreditation of EEG Technology Training Programs. Graduates of these programs receive associate's degrees or certificates.

Potential and Advancement There are about 6,400 EEG technologists, and this field is expected to grow rapidly through the year 2000. Greater acceptance of the value of the EEG and the willingness of health insurers to pay for this type of test will contribute to this growth. Opportunities for those with training in EEG technology should be excellent.

EEG technologists in hospital settings may advance by becoming chief EEG technologists, taking on more management and training responsibilities.

Income EEG technologists have average annual starting salaries of $15,924. More experienced technologists earn yearly salaries up to $27,360. Those in supervisory or training positions usually command higher salaries.

Additional Sources of Information

Executive Office
American Society of Electroneurodiagnostic Technologists Inc.
Sixth at Quint
Carroll, IA 51401

Joint Review Committee for the Accreditation of EEG Technology
   Training Programs
11526 53d Street, N
Clearwater, FL 34620

Emergency Medical Technician

The Job   Emergency medical technicians, or EMTs, are usually the first caregivers to arrive on the scene of a medical emergency. Their ability to provide medical care quickly and accurately may save a victim's life.

Upon arrival at the scene, EMTs must assess the situation and decide which emergency services must be given first. They must determine the victim's condition as well as whether he or she has any preexisting medical conditions, such as epilepsy or diabetes, that will affect the type of treatment given. Some of the medical treatments EMTs are trained to give include opening airways, restoring breathing, controlling breathing, treatment for shock, administering oxygen, assisting in childbirth, and treating and resuscitating heart attack victims.

Sometimes when a situation is very serious, EMTs must report directly to the hospital by radio, transmitting vital signs and other information, so that the hospital can then provide instructions for treatment.

Another difficulty EMTs sometimes face is that they must free trapped victims, as in a car accident or a collapsed building. They must somehow free the victim while making sure that he or she is not injured further.

If victims must be transported to the hospital, EMTs put them on stretchers, carry them to the ambulance, and place them inside, making sure that the stretcher is secure. One EMT drives the ambulance while the other stays with the victim and continues medical treatment. After the ambulance arrives at the hospital, the EMTs help get the victim into the emergency room and inform the physicians and nurses of their observations and the treatment they have given.

It is also the EMTs' responsibility to make sure that the ambulance is properly equipped and maintained. They must see that any supplies that have been used are either replaced or cleaned and sterilized and check the equipment to ensure that it is working properly. They also must see that the ambulance is in good working condition.

There are three classifications for EMTs: EMT-ambulance (EMT-A), EMT-intermediate, and EMT-paramedic. EMT-A's are basic EMTs. EMT-intermediates and EMT-paramedics have received more training and are capable of giving additional types of medical treatment. A fourth level—EMT-defibrillator (EMT-D)—is emerging. These EMTs are trained in using electrical defibrillation to resuscitate heart attack victims.

Places of Employment and Working Conditions

EMTs are employed by private ambulance services; hospitals; and municipal police, fire, and rescue squad departments.

EMTs work inside and outside, sometimes in poor weather conditions. EMTs' services are needed 24 hours a day, so they are often required to work evenings, weekends, and holidays. This job is physically strenuous—it involves a great deal of lifting. There is also much pressure in this field—EMTs must make life-and-death decisions as part of their regular job.

Qualifications, Education, and Training

EMTs must be physically strong and healthy. They must be able to make good decisions quickly in stressful situations. They should be emotionally stable and have leadership abilities. EMTs should have a neat and clean appearance and a pleasant personality.

EMTs are required to undergo instruction in emergency medical care techniques. The U.S. Department of Transportation has designed a national standard training program. The course is 110 hours long and trains EMT-A's in basic life support techniques. It is offered in all 50 states, the District of Columbia, and the Virgin Islands. The course is offered by police, fire, and health departments; hospitals; and medical schools, colleges, and universities.

Those taking the course learn how to deal with emergencies such as bleeding, fractures, oxygen administration, airway obstruction, cardiac arrest, and emergency childbirth.

After completing this course, students may take a two-day course in removing trapped victims and a five-day course in driving emergency vehicles.

To become an EMT-intermediate, EMT-A's must take additional courses and learn more medical procedures. EMT-paramedics have completed a nine-month training program to achieve their designation.

Applicants to EMT training courses must be at least 18 years old, have a high school diploma or its equivalent, and a valid driver's license.

The National Registry of Emergency Medical Technicians registers EMT-paramedics to meet its standards. While registration is not a requirement, it does give greater credibility to EMTs who have earned it.

All 50 states have certification procedures.

Potential and Advancement

There are currently 76,000 EMTs. There will be some growth in employment through the year 2000. The rapid growth in the number of senior citizens and developments in the field of emergency medicine will create a demand for EMTs. However, the high cost of training and equipping EMTs may lessen opportunities. The best job prospects will be with municipal governments and private ambulance services.

EMTs who have advanced through the ranks to become EMT-paramedics must leave fieldwork to advance any further. They may become field supervisor, operations supervisor, operations manager, administrative director, and then executive director.

Another advancement route for EMTs is to become an instructor, but this usually requires a bachelor's degree in education.

Other EMTs leave the field altogether, becoming sales representatives for emergency medical equipment manufacturers. Others become police officers or firefighters. By getting more education, some are able to move into clinical or management careers in health or related fields.

Income   Earnings for EMTs depend on the level of their experience and training, the type of employer they have, and their geographical area.

Average starting salaries for EMT-A's are $16,960 a year; for EMT-intermediates, $17,130; and EMT-paramedics, $22,510.

Additional Sources of Information

National Association of Emergency Medical Technicians
9140 Ward Parkway
Kansas City, MO 64114

National Registry of Emergency Medical Technicians
P.O. Box 29233
Columbus, OH 43229

Health Services Manager

The Job   The exact title may vary from institution to institution, but the responsibilities are the same—to plan, organize, coordinate, and supervise the delivery of health care. There are two types of health services managers: generalists, who manage or help to manage an entire facility; and health specialists, who manage specific clinical departments or services found only in the health industry.

The top administrator must staff the hospital with both medical and nonmedical personnel; provide all aspects of patient care services; purchase supplies and equipment; plan space allocations; and arrange for housekeeping items such as laundry, security, and maintenance. The administrator must also provide and work within a budget; act as liaison between the directors of the hospital and the medical staff; keep up with developments in the health care field including government regulations; handle hospital community relations; and sometimes act as a fund raiser.

In large facilities, the administrator has a staff of assistants with expertise in a variety of fields, but, in small- and medium-sized institutions, the administrator is responsible for all of them.

Health specialists manage the daily operations of individual, specialized departments such as surgery, rehabilitation therapy, nursing, and medical records. These workers have more narrowly defined responsibilities than generalists. They also receive more specialized training and experience in their field.

In addition to working in hospitals, health services managers are employed by nursing homes and extended care facilities, community health centers, mental health centers, outreach clinics, city or county health departments, and HMOs. Others are employed as advisors and specialists by insurance companies, government regulatory agencies, and professional standards organizations such as the American Cancer Society and the American Heart Association. Some serve as commissioned officers in the medical service and hospitals of the various armed forces or work for the U.S. Public Health Service or the Department of Veterans Affairs.

Depending on the size of the institution, a new graduate might start as an administrative assistant, an assistant administrator, a specialist in a specific management area, a department head, or an assistant department head. In a small health care facility, the new graduate would start in a position with broad responsibilities, while in a large hospital the position might be narrow in scope with rotating work in several departments necessary to gain broad experience.

Places of Employment and Working Conditions

Health services managers work throughout the country in hospitals and health care facilities of all sizes.

Health services managers put in long hours. They are on call at all times for emergency situations that affect the functioning of the institutions. They have very heavy workloads and are constantly under a great deal of pressure.

Qualifications, Education, and Training

Health services managers should have health and vitality, maturity, sound judgment, tact, patience, the ability to motivate others, good communication skills, and sensitivity for people.

Good grades in high school are important. Courses should include English, science, mathematics, business, public speaking, and social studies. Volunteer work or a part-time job in a hospital is helpful.

Preparation for this career includes the completion of an academic program in health administration that leads to a bachelor's, master's, or Ph.D. degree. The various levels of degree programs offer different levels of career preparation. Most health care organizations prefer to hire administrators with at least a master's degree in health administration, hospital administration, public health, or business administration. Usually, larger organizations require more academic preparation for their administrative positions.

The administrators of nursing homes must be licensed. Licensing requirements vary from state to state, but all require a specific level of education and experience.

Potential and Advancement There are about 177,000 people working in some phase of health care administration. Significant growth is projected for this field through the year 2000 as the increasing number of people 85 years old and over create a greater demand for health services.

The most opportunities will be in hospitals as well as in hospital subsidiaries that provide services such as ambulatory surgery, alcohol and drug abuse rehabilitation, hospice facilities, physicians' offices, outpatient care facilities, health and allied services, and nursing and long-term care facilities.

In spite of the tremendous growth in this field, there will be keen competition for upper-level management jobs in hospitals.

Health services managers advance as they move into higher paying positions with more responsibilities. They also may advance by transferring to another health care facility or organization.

Income Average earnings for all health services managers are $30,524 per year. Those at the low end of the salary range earn less than $15,704, while those at the high end earn an annual average of more than $50,800. Salaries vary depending on the manager's level of experience and expertise, the type and size of health facility, the geographic location, and the type of ownership.

Additional Sources of Information

American College of Health Care Administrators
8120 Woodmont Avenue
Suite 200
Bethesda, MD 20814

American College of Healthcare Executives
840 North Lake Shore Drive
Chicago, IL 60611

Association of University Programs in Health Administration
1911 Fort Myer Drive
Suite 503
Arlington, VA 22209

Medical Assistant

The Job Medical assistants perform administrative tasks and work with patients, helping doctors keep their practices running efficiently.

Medical assistants' duties vary from office to office, depending on the size of the medical practice. In smaller practices, they have a wider range of responsibilities, often performing both administrative and clinical tasks. In larger practices, they may specialize in a particular area.

Laws regarding the procedures medical assistants are permitted to perform vary from state to state, but some of the more common clinical tasks they are allowed to do include taking and recording medical histories and vital signs; explaining treatments to patients; preparing patients for examination; and assisting in examinations.

After an examination, medical assistants may collect laboratory specimens and perform basic laboratory tests; dispose of contaminated supplies; and sterilize medical instruments.

Some of the administrative duties medical assistants often have include answering telephones, greeting patients, recording and filing medical records, filling out insurance forms, scheduling appointments, arranging for hospital admission and laboratory tests, and taking care of billing and bookkeeping.

Some medical assistants specialize in a certain branch of medicine such as podiatry or ophthalmology.

Places of Employment and Working Conditions Most medical assistants work in doctors' offices; some work in the offices of optometrists, podiatrists, and chiropractors. Others work in hospitals.

Medical assistants usually have a 40-hour workweek, which may include some weekend and evening hours.

Qualifications, Education, and Training
Medical assistants spend a great deal of time working with people, so they must be neat, pleasant, and courteous. They must be able to listen and follow doctors' instructions closely and also listen to patients' needs.

There are no formal education requirements for medical assistants, and many receive their training on the job. However, formal programs in medical assisting are offered at secondary and postsecondary levels in technical high schools, vocational schools, community and junior colleges, and universities. Most doctors prefer to hire medical assistants with formal training.

Two agencies accredit medical assisting programs: the American Medical Association's Committee on Allied Health Education and Accreditation (CAHEA) and the Accrediting Bureau of Health Education Schools (ABHES). These programs usually include course work in biological sciences and medical terminology and typing, transcription, recordkeeping, accounting, and insurance processing.

There are no general licensing requirements for medical assistants, but some states require passing a test or completing a course for medical assistants who perform certain procedures such as taking x-rays, drawing blood, or giving injections.

Several associations certify or register medical assistants who meet their requirements. Employers often prefer to hire those who are certified and have experience.

Potential and Advancement
There are about 149,000 medical assistants. Job opportunities should be very good through the year 2000 due to the increasing demands for medical care.

Opportunities will be excellent for those with formal training, experience, or both. Those who are certified and have computer and word processing skills will have even greater advantages when seeking employment.

Medical assistants may advance by becoming office managers. Others become consultants for medical office management or for the medical insurance industry. Some work for hospitals as ward clerks, medical record clerks, phlebotomists, and EKG technicians. Others sometimes get further education and become nurses or work in some field of medical technology.

Income
Earnings for medical assistants vary widely depending on the worker's credentials and level of experience, the size and location of the employer, and the number of hours worked. A survey by CAHEA shows that start-

ing salaries for graduates of medical assisting programs it accredits average about $13,000 annually.

Additional Sources of Information

The American Association of Medical Assistants
20 North Wacker Drive
Suite 1575
Chicago, IL 60606

Registered Medical Assistants of American Medical Technologists
710 Higgins Road
Park Ridge, IL 60068

Medical Laboratory Technologist

The Job Medical laboratory work often appeals to people who would like to work in the medical field but who are not necessarily interested in direct care of patients. Those who work in medical laboratories are involved in the analysis of blood, tissue samples, and body fluids. They use precision instruments, equipment, chemicals, and other materials to detect and diagnose diseases. In some instances, such as blood tests, they also gather the specimens to be analyzed.

The work of medical laboratory technologists is done under the direction of a pathologist (a physician who specializes in the causes and nature of disease) or other physician or scientist who specializes in clinical chemistry, microbiology, or other biological sciences.

Medical technologists, who have four years of training, usually perform a wide variety of tests in small laboratories; those in large laboratories usually specialize in a single area such as parasitology, blood banking, or hematology (study of blood cells). Some do research, develop laboratory techniques, or perform supervisory and administrative duties.

Medical laboratory technicians, who have two years of training, have much the same testing duties but do not have the in-depth knowledge of the technologists. Technicians may also specialize in a particular field but are not usually involved in administrative work.

Medical laboratory assistants have about one year of formal training. They assist the technologists and technicians in some routine tests and are generally responsible for the care and sterilization of laboratory equipment, including glassware and instruments, and do some recordkeeping.

Most technologists, technicians, and laboratory assistants work in hospital laboratories. Others work in physicians' offices, independent laboratories, blood banks, public health agencies and clinics, pharmaceutical firms, and research institutions. The federal government employs them in the U.S. Public Health Service, the armed forces, and the Department of Veterans Affairs.

Places of Employment and Working Conditions

Work in this field is available in all areas of the country, with the largest concentrations in the larger cities.

Medical laboratory personnel work a 40-hour week with night and weekend shifts if they are employed in a hospital. Laboratories are usually clean and well lighted and contain a variety of testing equipment and materials. Although unpleasant odors are sometimes present and the work involves the processing of specimens of many kinds of diseased tissue, few hazards exist because of careful attention to safety and sterilization procedures.

Qualifications, Education, and Training

A strong interest in science and the medical field is essential. Manual dexterity, good eyesight, and normal color vision are necessary. One must also show attention to detail and accuracy and have the ability to work under pressure and the desire to take responsibility for his or her own work.

High school students interested in this field should take courses in science and mathematics and should select a training program carefully.

Medical technologists must have a college degree and complete a specialized program in medical technology. This specialized training is offered by hospitals and schools in programs accredited by either the Committee on Allied Health and Accreditation (CAHEA) in cooperation with the National Accrediting Agency for Clinical Laboratory Sciences (NAACLS) or the Accrediting Bureau of Health Education Schools (ABHES). The programs are usually affiliated with a college or university. A few training programs require a bachelor's degree for entry; others require only three years of college and award a bachelor's degree at the completion of the training program. Those who wish to specialize must complete an additional 12 months of study with extensive lab work.

Advanced degrees in this field are offered by many universities and are a plus for anyone interested in teaching, research, or administration.

Technicians may receive training in two-year educational programs in junior colleges, in two-year courses at four-year colleges and universities, in vocational and technical schools, or in the armed forces.

Medical laboratory assistants usually receive on-the-job training. Some hospitals—and junior colleges and vocational schools in conjunction with a

Medical Laboratory Technologist

hospital—also conduct one-year training programs, some of which are accredited by the ABHES. A high school diploma or equivalency diploma is necessary.

Medical technologists may be certified by the Board of Registry of the American Society of Clinical Pathologists, the American Medical Technologists, the National Certification Agency for Medical Laboratory Personnel, or the Credentialing Commission of the International Society of Clinical Laboratory Technology. These same organizations also certify technicians.

Some states require technologists and technicians to be licensed. This usually takes the form of a written examination. Other states often require registration.

Potential and Advancement There are about 242,000 persons employed as medical laboratory workers. Medical laboratory technology is a good job opportunity field since, like the entire medical field, it is expected to grow steadily due to population growth and the increase in prepaid medical insurance programs. Job opportunities will probably be slightly better for technicians and assistants, because the increasing use of automated lab equipment will allow them to perform tests that previously required technologists. Technologists will be needed for supervisory and administrative positions, however, and will continue to be in demand in laboratories where their level of training is required by state regulations or employer preference.

Advancement depends on education and experience. Assistants can advance to the position of technician or technologist by completing the required education; technicians can advance to supervisory positions or complete the required education for technologists. Advancement to administrative positions is usually limited to technologists.

Income Salaries in this field vary depending on employer and geographic location; the highest salaries are paid in the larger cities.

Newly graduated medical technologists start at about $20,000 a year; technicians at about $16,800. Experienced medical technologists earn an average of about $29,000 a year.

Additional Sources of Information

Accrediting Bureau of Health Education Schools
Oak Manor Office
29089 U.S. 20 West
Elkhart, IN 46514

American Medical Technologists
710 Higgins Road
Park Ridge, IL 60068

American Society of Clinical Pathologists
Board of Registry
P.O. Box 12270
Chicago, IL 60612

American Society for Medical Technology
2021 L Street, NW
Washington, DC 20036

International Society for Clinical Laboratory Technology
818 Olive Street
St. Louis, MO 63101

Medical Record Technician

The Job Medical record technicians are responsible for keeping an accurate permanent file on patients treated by doctors and hospitals.

When patients are undergoing treatment, doctors and hospitals keep records of their medical history, results of physical exams, x-ray and lab test reports, diagnoses and treatments, and doctors' and nurses' notes. Also included is information about the patients' symptoms, the tests undergone, and the response to treatment.

Medical record technicians assemble, organize, and check these records for completeness and accuracy. Often doctors and nurses record their information and observations on computer, and medical record technicians must retrieve them from the hospital's central computer.

After medical record technicians have gathered all of the information, they consult classification manuals and assign codes to the diagnoses and procedures included in the record. They then assign the patient to a diagnosis-related group (DRG), which determines the amount the hospital will be reimbursed by Medicare or other insurance programs that use the DRG system.

The medical records that technicians keep serve several important purposes. They are also important for documentation in the case of legal actions and for insurance claims and Medicare reimbursement.

Medical record technicians sometimes analyze data and provide statistics that help hospital administrators and planners keep the hospital running efficiently.

Medical Record Technician

Medical record technicians also sometimes collect and interpret medical records for law firms, insurance companies, government agencies, researchers, and patients.

Places of Employment and Working Conditions

Most medical record technicians work in hospitals; others work in medical group practices, HMOs, nursing homes, clinics, and other facilities that deliver health care.

Medical record technicians usually work a 40-hour week, with some overtime. Often they work day, evening, or night shifts because hospital medical record offices operate 18 to 24 hours a day.

Medical record technicians usually work in comfortable environments, but the work can be stressful because of the necessity for accuracy and close attention to detail.

Qualifications, Education, and Training

Medical record technicians who have earned the credential *accredited record technician* are generally preferred by employers. To become accredited, medical record technicians must pass a written examination given by the American Medical Record Association (AMRA). The requirement for taking the test is the completion of a two-year associate's degree program accredited by the Committee on Allied Health Education and Accreditation in collaboration with AMRA or the independent study program in medical record technology along with 30 semester hours in prescribed areas.

Medical record technology programs include course work in the biological sciences, medical terminology, medical record science, business management, legal aspects, and introduction to computer data processing.

Potential and Advancement

There are about 47,000 medical record technicians, and opportunities should be excellent for those who have completed a formal training program through the year 2000, primarily because of the important role they play in managing health care costs.

There are three major routes for advancement for medical record technicians—teaching, managing, or specializing. Experienced technicians who have a master's degree in a related field sometimes go into teaching. They can also advance into the management of a medical record department. Finally, technicians can advance into a specialty such as Medicare coding and tumor registry.

Income Medical record technicians earn an annual median salary of $17,200, according to the *Hospital and Health Care Report*.

Additional Source of Information

American Medical Record Association
875 North Michigan Avenue
John Hancock Center
Suite 1850
Chicago, IL 60611

Medical Secretary

The Job Secretaries are the center of communication in an office. The duties they perform keep offices running efficiently. Medical secretaries are specialized secretaries who are employed by physicians or medical scientists.

Medical secretaries transcribe dictation, type letters, and help doctors or medical scientists prepare reports, speeches, and articles.

They also have responsibilities similar to other secretaries. They take shorthand, deal with visitors, keep track of appointments, make travel arrangements, and see that any of the employer's paperwork is taken care of.

Places of Employment and Working Conditions Medical secretaries are employed throughout the country, in physicians' offices, hospitals, and other types of health agencies.

Working conditions vary, but full-time medical secretaries usually work a 37- to 40-hour week.

Qualifications, Education, and Training Medical secretaries must be accurate and neat. They must display discretion and initiative and have a good command of spelling, grammar, punctuation, and vocabulary. They need to know medical terms and be familiar with hospital or laboratory procedures.

High school business courses are valuable and so are college preparatory courses because secretaries should have a good general background. They should take as many English courses as possible.

Secretarial training as part of a college education or at a private business school is preferred by many employers. Training for specialty areas such as medicine can take a year or two.

Well-trained and highly experienced secretaries may qualify for the designation *certified professional secretary* (CPS) by passing a series of examinations given by the National Secretaries Association. This is a mark of achievement in the secretarial field and is recognized as such by many employers.

Potential and Advancement The demand for well-qualified medical secretaries will continue to grow as demand for medical services increases. Job opportunities should be very good through the year 2000.

Opportunities for advancement depend on the acquisition of new or improved skills and on increasing knowledge of the medical field. Some medical secretaries may become administrative assistants or office managers.

Income Salaries for medical secretaries vary greatly depending on the level of their skill, experience, and responsibility; the area of the country in which they work; and the type of employer they have.

The average annual salary for all types of secretaries is $21,710, with a range from $17,810 to $29,354. Secretaries working in the West and Midwest earn higher salaries in general than those working in the Northeast and South.

Additional Source of Information

Professional Secretaries International
301 East Armour Boulevard
Kansas City, MO 64111

Nuclear Medicine Technologist

The Job In nuclear medicine, radiation is used in the diagnosis and treatment of disease. Radiation, in the form of drugs called radiopharmaceuticals, is injected into patients or taken orally and is traced from outside the body to the organs or tissues where it settles in order to determine any of their abnormalities. Nuclear medicine technologists are the specially trained workers who perform these tests under the direction of a physician.

Nuclear medicine technologists must prepare the correct dosage of the radiopharmaceutical and administer it to the patient orally, by injection, or by other means. They must be careful in preparing the radiopharmaceutical to keep the radiation dose to workers and the patient as low as possible.

Once the radiopharmaceutical has entered the patient's system, the technologist uses diagnostic imaging equipment to trace and photograph the radiopharmaceutical as it passes through or settles in parts of the patient's body. After the test has been completed, the technologist views the images on film or on a computer screen to find any additional information to give to the physician, who will interpret the test results.

Although most of their time is spent working directly with patients, nuclear medicine technologists also perform laboratory tests and some administrative work, which involves keeping complete and accurate records.

Places of Employment and Working Conditions

Most nuclear medicine technologists hold jobs in hospitals, but a small number work in medical laboratories, physicians' offices, outpatient clinics, and imaging centers.

Nuclear medicine technologists typically work a 40-hour week. They may be required to work evening or night shifts and may be on call on a rotation basis.

The job can be physically demanding at times. Technologists spend a great deal of time on their feet, and they may have to lift or turn disabled patients.

If workers follow proper safety precautions and wear protective devices, the danger of radiation exposure is minimal. Technologists wear special badges that measure the level of radiation in the area they are working. This measurement very rarely approaches or exceeds established safety levels.

Qualifications, Education, and Training

In the past, training was typically given on the job. Now, however, employers prefer to hire technologists who have completed formal training programs. These programs are offered in hospitals, community colleges, universities, and Department of Veterans Affairs medical centers. It is important to realize that there are several different types of programs; they differ in length, prerequisites, class size, cost, and degree awarded upon completion. Another important factor to consider in selecting a program is whether it is accredited by the Committee on Allied Health Education and Accreditation (CAHEA). There are 106 CAHEA-accredited programs currently. Many hospitals will hire only those who have completed one of these programs.

Nuclear Medicine Technologist

One-year programs are offered to those who already have some experience in health care or a science background, such as medical technologists, registered nurses, or respiratory therapists. Graduates are granted a certificate.

Those with no previous training in health care may choose a two-year certificate program; a two-year associate's degree program; or a four-year baccalaureate program.

Licensure is required in seven states and Puerto Rico. Voluntary certification or registration is available from the American Registry of Radiologic Technologists (ARRT) and the Nuclear Medicine Technology Certification Board (NMTCB). Some employers will give greater consideration to technologists with these credentials.

Potential and Advancement There are currently over 10,000 nuclear medicine technologists. The nuclear medicine technology field is expected to grow faster than the average for all occupations through the year 2000. Excellent employment opportunities exist, and there are reports of a shortage of technologists in this field as enrollment in accredited training programs declines.

Technologists may advance by becoming supervisors or by specializing in an area such as computer analysis or nuclear cardiology. Some technologists become instructors or directors of nuclear medicine technology programs. Others may work in research. Some leave the occupation and become sales representatives with health equipment manufacturing firms or radiopharmaceutical companies or work as radiation safety officers.

Income Salaries for beginning technologists average about $20,820 a year. More experienced technologists earn, on average, about $27,012.

Additional Sources of Information

American Society of Radiologic Technologists
1500 Central Avenue
Albuquerque, NM 87123

Division of Allied Health Education and Accreditation
American Medical Association
535 North Dearborn Street
Chicago, IL 60610

The Society of Nuclear Medicine
136 Madison Avenue
New York, NY 10016

Nurse, Licensed Practical

The Job Licensed practical nurses (LPNs) provide much of the bedside care for patients in hospitals, nursing homes, and extended care facilities. They work under the direction of physicians and registered nurses and perform duties that require technical knowledge but not the professional education and training of a registered nurse. In some areas they are called licensed vocational nurses.

LPNs take and record temperatures and blood pressures, change dressings, administer certain prescribed medicine, bathe patients, care for newborn infants, and perform some special nursing procedures.

Those who work in private homes provide daily nursing care and sometimes prepare meals for the patient as well. LPNs employed in physicians' offices or clinics may perform some clerical chores and handle appointments.

Places of Employment and Working Conditions

Licensed practical nurses work in all areas of the country, most of them in hospitals.

LPNs usually work a 40-hour week, but since patients require 24-hour care, they may work some nights, weekends, and holidays. They spend most of their working hours on their feet and help patients move in bed, stand, or walk. They also experience the stress of working with sick patients and their families.

LPNs face many hazards and difficulties on their jobs. They often come into contact with caustic chemicals, radiation, and infectious diseases. They may also suffer from back injuries and muscle strains when moving patients. The people they take care of may often be confused, angry, or depressed.

Qualifications, Education, and Training

Anyone interested in working as a practical nurse should have a concern for the sick, be emotionally stable, and have physical stamina. The ability to follow orders and work under close supervision is also necessary.

A high school diploma is not always necessary for enrollment in a training program, although it is usually preferred. One-year, state-approved programs are offered by trade, technical, and vocational schools; high schools; junior colleges; local hospitals; health agencies; and private institutions. Some army training programs are also state approved.

Applicants for state licensing must complete a program in practical nursing that has been approved by the state board of nursing and must pass a written examination.

Nurse, Registered

Potential and Advancement There are about 626,000 licensed practical nurses. The employment outlook for LPNs is very good through the next decade.

Advancement in this field is limited without formal education or additional training. Training programs in some hospitals help LPNs complete the educational requirements necessary to become registered nurses while they continue to work part-time.

Income Starting salaries for LPNs working in hospitals average about $15,900 a year. Experienced LPNs average about $21,400 a year.

Additional Sources of Information

Communications Department
National League for Nursing
350 Hudson Street
New York, NY 10014

National Association for Practical Nurse Education and Service, Inc.
1400 Spring Street
Suite 310
Silver Spring, MD 20910

National Federation of Licensed Practical Nurses, Inc.
P.O. Box 1088
Raleigh, NC 27619

Nurse, Registered

The Job Registered nurses (RNs) play a major role in health care. As part of a health care team, they administer medications and treatments as prescribed by a physician, provide skilled bedside nursing care for the sick and the injured, and work toward the prevention of illness and the promotion of good health.

Most nurses are employed in hospitals where they usually work with a group of patients requiring similar care such as a postsurgery floor, the children's area (pediatrics), or the maternity section. Some specialize in operating room work.

Doctors, dentists, and oral surgeons employ nurses in their offices to perform routine laboratory and office work in addition to nursing duties. Industries employ nurses to assist with health examinations, treat minor injuries of employees, and arrange for further medical care if it is necessary. Industrial nurses may also do some recordkeeping and handle claims for medical insurance and workers' compensation.

Community health nurses work with patients in their homes, schools, public health clinics, and in other community settings. Nurses also teach in nursing schools and conduct continuing education courses for registered and licensed practical nurses.

Private duty nurses are self-employed nurses who provide individual care in hospitals or homes for one patient at a time when the patient needs constant attention. This care may be required for just a short time or for extended periods.

Registered nurses who receive special advanced training may become *nurse practitioners*. They are permitted to perform some services, such as physical examinations, that have been traditionally handled by physicians. Nurse practitioners are an important part of many neighborhood health center staffs.

The federal government employs nurses in Veterans Administration hospitals and clinics, in the U.S. Public Health Service, and as commissioned officers in the armed forces.

Most nurses are women, but young men are entering the field in increasing numbers in recent years.

Places of Employment and Working Conditions

Nurses are usually on their feet most of the day. Those who work in hospitals, nursing homes, or as private duty nurses must be prepared to work evenings, weekends, and holidays.

Nurses need both physical and emotional stamina to cope with the stresses of their jobs. They face the dangers of infectious diseases and the hazards of working with radiation, chemicals, and gases. They also must be careful to avoid back injuries and muscle strains when moving patients.

Qualifications, Education, and Training

Nurses need the ability to follow orders precisely, use good judgment in emergencies, and cope with human suffering, and they must have good physical and emotional stamina.

In high school, students should take a college preparation program with an emphasis on science.

There are three types of training for registered nurses. Many hospitals offer three-year diploma programs in their own nursing schools that combine classroom instruction and clinical experience within the hospital. Four-year bachelor degree programs are available at many colleges. Two-year associate degree programs are offered by some junior and community colleges. These degree pro-

Nurse, Registered

grams are combined with clinical practice in an affiliated hospital or health care facility.

A bachelor's degree is required for administrative or management positions in nursing; research, teaching, and clinical specializations usually require a master's degree.

Potential and Advancement

There are about 1,577,000 registered nurses, one-fourth of them working part-time. Future employment opportunities should be excellent for some time due to a current shortage of nurses. Nursing opportunities exist in every community; there are shortages of qualified nurses in many inner-city areas and in some southern states. Employment prospects for nurses with specialized training in fields such as intensive care, geriatrics, and oncology are excellent.

Experienced hospital nurses can advance to head nurse or assistant director or director of nursing services. Many supervisory and management positions require a bachelor's degree, however.

Income

Registered nurses working in hospitals start at average annual salaries of about $23,100. Experienced nurses earn an average of about $32,100, while experienced head nurses average about $40,800. Nurses working in nursing homes have a median annual salary of about $21,300.

Additional Sources of Information

American Nurses' Association
2420 Pershing Road
Kansas City, MO 64108

Communications Department
National League for Nursing
350 Hudson Street
New York, NY 10014

Nursing Aide

The Job Nursing aides, also called nursing assistants or hospital attendants, provide care for patients in hospitals and in long-term care facilities such as nursing homes. Working under the supervision of registered and licensed practical nurses, they perform some of the more routine patient care duties.

Hospital nursing aides' tasks include taking patients' temperature, pulse, and blood pressure; helping patients in and out of bed; escorting them to operating and examining rooms; and feeding, dressing, and bathing them. They also make beds, serve meals, and move supplies.

Nursing aides in nursing homes have a great deal of contact with patients—far more than other members of the staff. They are the primary caregivers and perform many of the same tasks as hospital nursing aides.

Places of Employment and Working Conditions Almost half of all nursing aides work in nursing homes, and others work in hospitals and state and county mental institutions.

Full-time nursing aides usually work 40 hours a week or less. Because patients need round-the-clock care, their work hours may include evenings, nights, weekends, and holidays.

This job is physically demanding and includes some unpleasant tasks. Workers spend a great deal of time on their feet and may have to move patients who are paralyzed or help them get in and out of bed, stand, and walk. Job duties include emptying bed pans, changing soiled bed linens, and caring for depressed or irritated patients.

Qualifications, Education, and Training Nursing aides must want to help people; they need to be patient, understanding, emotionally stable, and dependable.

Most employers require neither a high school diploma nor prior work experience. Some hospitals require work experience, and some nursing homes require aides to complete 75 hours of mandatory training and pass a written exam within four months of employment. This is a good field for young people to gain exposure to health care occupations since many employers accept applicants who are 17 or 18 years old.

There are some training programs for nursing aides in high schools, vocational-technical centers, and some nursing homes and community colleges.

Potential and Advancement There are about 1,184,000 nursing aides, and job prospects through the year 2000 are excellent. Because of the growing elderly population, nursing aides will find jobs primarily in the growing number of nursing homes. Also nursing aides will be needed to care for the growing number of people whose lives are saved due to advanced medical technology but who never fully recover.

There are very limited opportunities for advancement in this field. There may be job opportunities for nursing aides who take additional training in a health care occupation.

Income Annual earnings for full-time nursing aides range from $7,000 to $21,100 or more, with the median earnings being about $11,500.

Additional Sources of Information

American Health Care Association
1201 L Street, NW
Washington, DC 20005

American Hospital Association
Division of Nursing
840 North Lake Shore Drive
Chicago, IL 60611

Occupational Therapist

The Job This fast-growing field offers personal satisfaction as well as financially rewarding job opportunities. Occupational therapists work with both the physically and emotionally disabled, helping some to return to normal functions and activities and others to make the fullest use of whatever talents they may have.

Occupational therapists plan and direct educational, vocational, and recreational activities; evaluate capabilities and skills; and plan individual therapy programs, often working as part of a medical team. Their clients are all ages and can range from a stroke victim relearning daily routines such as eating, dressing, and using a telephone to an accident victim learning to reuse impaired limbs before returning to work.

To restore mobility and dexterity to hands disabled by injury or disease, occupational therapists teach manual and creative skills through the use of crafts such as weaving, knitting, and leather working. They design games and activities especially for children or make special equipment or splints to aid the disabled patient.

Many part-time positions are available for occupational therapists; some occupational therapists work for more than one employer, traveling between job locations and clients.

In addition to hospital rehabilitation departments, other types of organizations that employ occupational therapists are rehabilitation centers and nursing homes, schools, mental health centers, schools and camps for handicapped children, state health departments and home care programs, Department of Veterans Affairs hospitals and clinics, psychiatric centers, and schools for learning and developmental disabilities.

Most occupational therapists are women, but the number of men entering the field has been increasing. Because there are many opportunities for part-time work, this is a good field for people with family responsibilities.

Related jobs are physical therapist and respiratory therapist.

Places of Employment and Working Conditions

Occupational therapists usually work a 40-hour week, but this may include weekends and evenings. Those who work for schools have regular school hours.

Therapists spend a lot of time on their feet, and they may be subject to back injuries and muscle strains from lifting and moving patients and equipment. Therapists who give home health care may spend several hours a day driving.

Qualifications, Education, and Training

Maturity, patience, imagination, manual skills, and the ability to instruct are important as is a sympathetic but objective attitude toward illness and disability.

Anyone considering this career field should have high school science courses, especially biology and chemistry. Courses in health and social studies along with training in crafts are also important. Volunteer work or a summer job in a health care facility can provide valuable exposure to this field.

A bachelor's degree in occupational therapy is required to practice in this field. Thirty-four states, Puerto Rico, and the District of Columbia require a license. Sixty-three colleges and universities offer bachelor's degrees in occupational therapy.

Occupational Therapist

Some schools offer a shorter program leading to certification or to a master's degree in occupational therapy for students who already have a bachelor's degree in another field.

Occupational therapy students study physical, biological, and behavioral sciences as well as the application of occupational therapy and skills. Students also spend from six to nine months working in hospitals or health agencies to gain clinical experience.

Graduates of accredited programs take the certification examination of the American Occupational Therapy Association to become a registered occupational therapist (OTR).

Potential and Advancement   There are about 33,000 occupational therapists with approximately 40 percent employed in hospitals. Employment in this field is expected to grow substantially because the public is becoming more interested and more knowledgeable about programs for rehabilitating the disabled. Job opportunities will be excellent on the whole through the year 2000; however, as the increasing number of qualified graduates catches up to the number of available jobs, competition for job openings may develop in some geographic areas.

Advancement in this field is usually to supervisory or administrative positions. Advanced education is necessary for those wishing to teach, do research, or advance to top administration levels.

Income   Beginning therapists employed by hospitals average about $24,000 a year; experienced therapists earn an average of $31,800.

Additional Source of Information

American Occupational Therapy Association
P.O. Box 1725
1383 Piccard Drive
Rockville, MD 29850-4375

Ophthalmic Laboratory Technician

The Job After an optometrist or ophthalmologist has examined a patient's eyes and prescribed corrective lenses, the prescription is sent to a laboratory where an ophthalmic laboratory technician, also called a manufacturing optician, optical mechanic, or optical goods worker, makes the lenses according to specifications and fits them into frames to produce finished glasses.

The order sent by the optometrist or ophthalmologist specifies the degree of curvature of the lens that will improve the patient's vision. The technician marks on a blank lens where the curves should be ground, sets the dials on a lens grinder for the correct degree of curvature, and starts and monitors the machine. After the lens has been ground, the technician finishes it by smoothing out the rough edges and polishing it.

The technician then uses special equipment to make sure the lenses meet the specifications on the prescription. The lenses are then cut and beveled to fit the frame, and the technician assembles lenses and frame into a finished pair of glasses.

In small laboratories, a technician will handle each step in this process; in larger laboratories, technicians may specialize in one particular step.

Places of Employment and Working Conditions About half of all ophthalmic laboratory technicians work in retail stores that manufacture prescription glasses and sell them directly to the public. Most of the rest work in optical laboratories, and a few work for optometrists and ophthalmologists.

Most technicians work a 40-hour, five-day week, with some weekend and evening hours. Their working environment is usually clean, well lighted, and quiet. They may be required to stand most of the time.

Qualifications, Education, and Training Ophthalmic laboratory technicians must be detail oriented, able to follow instructions, and have good manual dexterity. Employers usually prefer to hire workers with a high school diploma.

Almost all technicians receive their training on the job, but there are a few formal programs in vocational-technical institutes and trade schools. Those trained on the job go through a 6- to 18-month training program, first learning the more basic tasks and gradually learning more difficult tasks.

Potential and Advancement There are currently about 26,000 ophthalmic laboratory technicians, and the field is expected to grow rapidly through the year 2000. Retail optical chains will offer the most new jobs.

Technicians usually advance by becoming supervisors or managers. Some receive further education and become dispensing opticians.

Income Most technicians earn between $10,000 and $15,000 a year. Trainees usually are paid minimum wage and are given increases as they gain skills.

Additional Source of Information

Commission on Opticianry Accreditation
10111 Martin Luther King, Jr., Highway
Suite 110
Bowie, MD 20715

Ophthalmologist

The Job Ophthalmologists are also called eye physician-surgeons. They are qualified physicians and osteopathic physicians who have completed additional specialized training in the treatment of eye diseases and disorders. They treat a full range of eye problems including vision deficiencies, injuries, infections, and other disorders with medicines, therapy, corrective lenses, or surgery. Their job is distinct from that of optometrists and opticians, who are not physicians and treat only vision problems.

Most ophthalmologists are in private practice. Others are employed by hospitals and clinics, medical schools and research foundations, federal and state agencies, and the armed forces.

Related jobs are optometrist, dispensing optician, physician, and osteopathic physician.

Places of Employment and Working Conditions Ophthalmologists work in all areas of the country. Those who are osteopathic physicians are concentrated in the areas that have osteopathic facilities—mainly in Florida, Michigan, Pennsylvania, New Jersey, Ohio, Texas, and Missouri. The workweek for ophthalmologists is from 35 to 50 hours. Those involved in general patient care are always on call for emergencies.

Qualifications, Education, and Training
Information on the training and licensing requirements for physicians and osteopathic physicians is contained in the appropriate job description elsewhere in this book.

An additional three to five years of residency in an accredited ophthalmology program must be completed by doctors who wish to specialize in this field. Candidates for the specialty must then pass the certification examination of the American Board of Ophthalmology or the American Osteopathic Board of Ophthalmology.

Potential and Advancement
The demand for ophthalmologists will continue to grow as the population grows. Greater interest in eye care, the growing number of senior citizens, and the increase in health insurance plans will all add to the need for qualified practitioners of this medical specialty.

Income
Ophthalmologists who start a private practice face a few lean years until the practice is established. In addition, a sizable investment in specialized equipment is necessary. Earnings during this early period may barely meet expenses.

As a practice grows, earnings usually increase substantially. Average annual earnings for all ophthalmologists are in the $75,000 range with some earning even more. In general, ophthalmologists in private practice earn more than those in salaried positions.

Additional Sources of Information

American Academy of Ophthalmology
655 Beach Street
P.O. Box 7424
San Francisco, CA 94120

American Medical Association
535 North Dearborn Street
Chicago, IL 60610

Optician, Dispensing

The Job   Over half the people in the United States use some form of corrective lenses (eyeglasses or contact lenses). These corrective lenses are prepared and fitted by dispensing opticians, who are also called ophthalmic dispensers. Working with the prescription received from an ophthalmologist (eye physician) or optometrist, the dispensing optician provides the customer with the appropriate eyeglasses. He or she measures the customer's face, aids in the selection of the appropriate frames, directs the work of ophthalmic laboratory technicians who grind the lenses, and fits the completed eyeglasses.

In many states, dispensing opticians also fit contact lenses, which requires even more skill, care, and patience than the preparation and fitting of eyeglasses. Opticians measure the corneas of the customer's eyes and, following the ophthalmologist's or optometrist's prescription, prepare specifications for the contact lens manufacturer. The optician will instruct the customer on how to insert, remove, and care for the contact lenses and will provide follow-up attention during the first few weeks.

Some dispensing opticians specialize in the fitting of artificial eyes and cosmetic shells to cover blemished eyes. Some also do their own lens grinding.

Most dispensing opticians work for retail optical shops or other retail stores with optical departments. Ophthalmologists and optometrists who sell glasses directly to patients also employ dispensing opticians, as do hospitals and eye clinics. A number of dispensing opticians operate their own retail shops and sell other optical goods such as binoculars, magnifying glasses, and sunglasses.

Places of Employment and Working Conditions   Dispensing opticians are located throughout the United States with most employed in large cities and in the more populous states. Working conditions are usually quiet and clean with a workweek of five or six days. Dispensing opticians who own their own businesses usually work longer hours than those employed by retail shops or by ophthalmologists and optometrists.

Qualifications, Education, and Training   The ability to do precision work is essential for anyone planning a career as a dispensing optician. Patience, tact, and the ability to deal with people are other valuable assets.

Applicants for entry-level jobs in this field need a high school diploma with courses in the basic sciences. High school courses in physics, algebra, geometry, and mechanical drawing are especially valuable.

Most opticians acquire their skills through on-the-job training. A small number of dispensing opticians learn their trade in the armed forces. In addition, large manufacturers of contact lenses offer nondegree courses in lensfitting.

Forty programs offer a two-year full-time course in optical fabricating and dispensing which leads to an associate's degree; 15 are accredited by the Commission on Opticianry Accreditation. Students learn optical mathematics, optical physics, and the use of precision measuring instruments.

Apprenticeship programs lasting from two to five years are also available. In these programs, the students study optometric technical subjects and basic office management and sales and work directly with patients in the fitting of eyeglasses and contact lenses.

Dispensing opticians must be licensed in at least 22 states. Specific requirements vary from state to state but generally include minimum standards of education and training along with a written or practical examination.

Potential and Advancement

About 49,000 persons work as dispensing opticians. Employment opportunities in this field are expected to grow steadily along with the population. Increased health insurance coverage, Medicare services, and state programs to provide eye care to low-income families—along with current fashion trends, which encourage sales of more than one pair of glasses to individual buyers—will add to the demand for dispensing opticians.

Many dispensing opticians go into business for themselves. Others advance to positions in the management of retail optical stores or become sales representatives for wholesalers or manufacturers of eyeglasses or contact lenses.

Income

Earnings for dispensing opticians vary a great deal. Highest earnings are in those states that require licensure. The average annual earnings for dispensing opticians are $25,000 a year and range from about $15,000 to $30,000.

Additional Sources of Information

National Academy of Opticianry
10111 Martin Luther King, Jr., Highway
Suite 112
Bowie, MD 20715

Opticians Association of America
10341 Democracy Lane
P.O. Box 10110
Fairfax, VA 22030

Optometrist

The Job Over half of the U.S. population wear corrective lenses (eyeglasses or contact lenses). Before obtaining lenses, people need an eye examination and a prescription to obtain the correct lenses for their particular eye problem. Optometrists (doctors of optometry) provide the bulk of this care.

In addition to handling vision problems, optometrists also check for disease. When evidence of disease is found, an optometrist refers the patient to the appropriate medical practitioner. Optometrists also check depth and color perception and the ability to focus and coordinate the eyes. They may prescribe corrective eye exercises or other treatments that do not require surgery. Optometrists can utilize medications for diagnosis, while in 23 states they can also treat eye diseases with drugs.

Some optometrists specialize in work with children or the aged or work only with the partially sighted who must wear microscopic or telescopic lenses. Industrial eye-safety programs also are an optometric specialty. A few optometrists are engaged in teaching and research.

Although most optometrists are in private practice, many others are in partnerships or in group practice with other optometrists or with other physicians as part of a health care team. Some work in retail vision chain stores. Many combine private, group, or partnership practice with work in specialized hospitals and eye clinics.

Some optometrists serve as commissioned officers in the armed forces. Others are consultants to engineers specializing in safety or lighting; to educators in remedial reading; and to health advisory committees of federal, state, and local governments.

Places of Employment and Working Conditions Although most optometrists work in California, Illinois, New York, Pennsylvania, and Ohio, opportunities exist in towns and cities of all sizes.

Most self-employed optometrists can set their own work schedule but often work longer than 40 hours a week. Because the work is not physically strenuous, optometrists can practice past the normal retirement age.

Qualifications, Education, and Training Because most optometrists are self-employed, anyone planning on a career in this field needs business ability and self-discipline in addition to the ability to deal effectively with people.

High school preparation should emphasize science, and business courses are also helpful.

The doctor of optometry degree is awarded after successful completion of at least six years of college. The two years of preoptometrical study should include English, mathematics, physics, chemistry, and biology or zoology. Some schools also require psychology, social studies, literature, philosophy, and foreign languages.

Admission to optometry schools is highly competitive. Because the number of qualified applicants exceeds the available places, applicants need superior grades in preoptometric courses to increase their chances of acceptance by one of the 16 schools of optometry approved by the Council on Optometric Education of the American Optometric Association.

Optometrists who wish to advance in a specialized field of optometry may study for a master's or Ph.D. degree in visual science, physiological optics, neurophysiology, public health, health administration, health information and communication, or health education. Career officers in the armed forces also have an opportunity to work toward advanced degrees and to do research.

Potential and Advancement There are about 37,000 practicing optometrists, many of them in private practice. Employment opportunities are expected to grow steadily through the year 2000. Increasing coverage of optometric services by health insurance, greater recognition of the importance of good vision, and the growing population—especially older people who are most likely to need eyeglasses—should contribute to an increase in the demand for optometrists.

Income Incomes for optometrists vary greatly depending on location, specialization, and factors such as private or group practice. New optometry graduates average $40,000 in their first year.

Experienced optometrists average about $65,000 a year with those in associate or partnership practices earning substantially more than those in private practice.

Additional Source of Information

American Optometric Association
243 North Lindbergh Boulevard
St. Louis, MO 63141

Osteopathic Physician

The Job   The dictionary defines osteopathy as "a system of medical practice based on the theory that diseases are due chiefly to a loss of structural integrity in the tissues and that this integrity can be restored by manipulation of the parts, supported by the use of medicines, surgery, proper diet, and other therapy."

Most osteopathic physicians are family doctors engaged in general practice. They see patients at the office or make house calls and treat patients in osteopathic and other private and public hospitals. Some osteopathic physicians specialize in such fields as internal medicine, neurology, psychiatry, ophthalmology, pediatrics, anesthesiology, physical medicine and rehabilitation, dermatology, obstetrics and gynecology, pathology, proctology, radiology, and surgery.

Most osteopathic physicians are in private practice, although a few hold salaried positions in private industry or government agencies. Others hold full-time positions with osteopathic hospitals and colleges where they are engaged in teaching, research, and writing.

Places of Employment and Working Conditions   Most osteopathic physicians practice in states that have osteopathic hospital facilities; over half are in Florida, Michigan, Pennsylvania, New Jersey, Ohio, Texas, and Missouri. Most general practitioners are located in towns and cities having less than 50,000 people; specialists are usually located in larger cities.

Qualifications, Education, and Training   Anyone interested in becoming an osteopathic physician should have emotional stability, patience, tact, and the interest and ability to deal effectively with people.

The education requirements for the doctor of osteopathy (D.O.) degree include a minimum of three years of college (although most applicants have a bachelor's degree) plus a three- to four-year professional program. The education and training of an osteopathic physician is very expensive due primarily to the length of time involved. Federal and private funds are available for loans, and federal scholarships are available to those who qualify and agree to a minimum of two years of service for the federal government after completion of training.

Undergraduate study must include courses in chemistry, physics, biology, and English, with high grades an important factor for acceptance into the professional programs. In addition to high grades, schools require a good score on the Medical College Admission Test (MCAT) and letters of recommendation. One very important qualification is the applicant's desire to study osteopathy rather than some other field of medicine.

During the first half of the professional program, the student studies basic sciences such as anatomy, physiology, and pathology as well as the principles of osteopathy. The second half of the program consists primarily of clinical experience. After graduation, a 12-month internship is usually completed at one of the osteopathic hospitals approved for internship or residency by the American Osteopathic Association. Those who intend to specialize must complete an additional two to five years of training.

All practicing osteopathic physicians must be licensed. State licensing requirements vary, but all states require graduation from an approved school of osteopathic medicine and a passing grade on a state board examination. Most states require an internship at an approved hospital.

Potential and Advancement There are about 53,500 practicing osteopathic physicians in the United States. Population growth, an increase in the number of persons covered by medical insurance, and the establishment of additional osteopathic hospitals will contribute to an increasing demand for osteopathic physicians. The greatest demand will continue to be in states where osteopathic medicine is well known and accepted as a form of treatment.

Opportunities for new practitioners are best in rural areas (many localities lack medical practitioners of any kind), small towns, and suburbs of large cities. The availability of osteopathic hospital facilities should be considered when one is selecting a location for practice.

Income As is usually the case in any field where setting up an individual practice is the norm, earnings in the first few years are low. Income usually rises substantially once the practice becomes established, and, in the case of osteopathic physicians, is very high in comparison with other professionals. Geographic location and the income level of the community are also factors that affect the level of income. The average annual income of general practitioners is $91,500.

Additional Sources of Information

American Association of Colleges of Osteopathic Medicine
6110 Executive Boulevard
Suite 405
Rockville, MD 20852

American Osteopathic Association
Department of Public Relations
142 East Ontario Street
Chicago, IL 60611

Pharmacist

The Job Pharmacists dispense drugs and medicines prescribed by physicians and dentists, advise on the use and proper dosage of prescription and nonprescription medicines, and work in research and marketing positions. Many pharmacists own their own businesses.

The majority of pharmacists work in community pharmacies (drugstores). These range from one-person operations to large retail establishments employing a staff of pharmacists.

Hospitals and clinics employ pharmacists to dispense drugs and medication to patients, advise the medical staff on the selection and effects of drugs, buy medical supplies, and prepare sterile solutions. In some hospitals, they also teach nursing classes.

Pharmaceutical manufacturers employ pharmacists in research and development and in sales positions. Drug wholesalers also employ them as sales and technical representatives.

The federal government employs pharmacists in hospitals and clinics of the Department of Veterans Affairs or the U.S. Public Health Service; in the Department of Defense; the Food and Drug Administration; the Department of Health, Education, and Welfare; and in the Drug Enforcement Administration. State and local health agencies also employ pharmacists.

Many community and hospital pharmacists also do consulting work for nursing homes and other health facilities that do not employ a full-time pharmacist.

Places of Employment and Working Conditions Just about every community has a drugstore employing at least one pharmacist. Most job opportunities, however, are in larger cities and densely populated metropolitan areas.

Pharmacists average about a 44-hour workweek; those who also do consulting work average an additional 15 hours a week. Pharmacists in community pharmacies work longer hours—including evenings and weekends—than those employed by hospitals and other health care institutions, pharmaceutical manufacturers, and drug wholesalers. Some community and hospital pharmacies are open around the clock; pharmacists employed by them may have to work nights, weekends, and holidays.

Qualifications, Education, and Training

Prospective pharmacists need an interest in medicine and should have orderliness and accuracy, business ability, honesty, and integrity.

Biology and chemistry courses along with some business courses should be taken in high school.

At least five years of study beyond high school are necessary to earn a degree in pharmacy. A few colleges admit pharmacy students immediately following high school, but most require one or two years of prepharmacy college and study in mathematics, basic sciences, humanities, and social sciences.

Seventy-four colleges of pharmacy are accredited by the American Council on Pharmaceutical Education. Most of these schools award a bachelor of science (B.S.) or a bachelor of pharmacy (B.Pharm.) degree upon completion of the required course of study. About one-third of the schools also offer an advanced degree program leading to a doctor of pharmacy (Pharm.D.) degree. A few schools offer only the Pharm.D. degree.

A Pharm.D. degree or a master's or Ph.D. degree in pharmacy or a related field is usually required for research, teaching, and administrative positions.

Pharmacists are usually required to serve an internship under the supervision of a registered pharmacist before they can obtain a license to practice. All states require a license and an applicant usually must have: 1) graduated from an accredited pharmacy college; 2) passed a state board of examination; and 3) had a specified amount of practical experience or internship. Many pharmacists are licensed to practice in more than one state, and most states will grant a license without examination to a qualified pharmacist licensed by another state.

Potential and Advancement

About 162,000 people work as pharmacists. Job opportunities are expected to be excellent through the year 2000 as the population becomes older and has more pharmaceutical needs. Shortages may even occur in states with high concentrations of the elderly.

Many pharmacists in salaried positions advance by opening their own community pharmacies. Those employed by chain drugstores may advance to management positions or executive-level jobs within the company. Hospital pharmacists may advance to director of pharmacy service or to other administrative positions.

Pharmacists employed by the pharmaceutical industry have the widest latitude of advancement possibilities because they can advance in management, sales, research, quality control, advertising, production, or packaging. There will be fewer job opportunities, however, with manufacturers than in other areas of pharmacy.

Pharmacologist

Income Experienced pharmacists working in chain drugstores earn an average of $41,800 a year; those working in independent drugstores earn an average of $38,200 a year; and hospital pharmacists average $42,600 a year.

Additional Sources of Information

American Association of Colleges of Pharmacy
1426 Prince Street
Alexandria, VA 22314

American Society of Hospital Pharmacists
4630 Montgomery Avenue
Bethesda, MD 20814

National Association of Boards of Pharmacy
1300 Higgins Road
Suite 103
Park Ridge, IL 60068

Pharmacologist

The Job Pharmacologists research the effects of drugs, chemicals, and other substances on humans and animals. The results of their research indicate how drugs and chemicals act at the cellular level; how drugs can best be used; appropriate drug dosages; the effects of materials such as chemicals, pesticides, and poisons; and dangerous substances and levels of chemicals.

In their laboratories, pharmacologists perform research, using live animals, plants, and human tissues. They sometimes inject chemicals or substances into animals or culture them with live tissue samples taken from animals or humans. The goal of their research is to determine the effects of these substances on organs and body systems and to identify any harmful side effects. After they have determined the positive and negative features of a drug, they can predict how useful a drug may be as a remedy for diseases, establish appropriate dosages, and inform doctors of how and when a drug should be used.

Pharmacologists often specialize in drugs affecting a particular organ or body system: *neuropharmacologists* focus on the nervous system; *cardiovascular pharmacologists,* cardiovascular and circulatory systems; *endocrine pharmacologists,* hormones; and *psychopharmacologists,* human and animal behavior.

Places of Employment and Working Conditions

Most pharmacologists work in modern laboratories in hospitals, research institutions, and pharmaceutical companies.

A 40-hour workweek is typical for most pharmacologists. The job requires a great deal of patience because experiments sometimes are not completed for weeks or even months. They sometimes face intense pressure to achieve results where loss of life may involve unexplained chemicals or other substances.

Qualifications, Education, and Training

Pharmacologists must have an aptitude for science. Patience is an important quality because research projects may take months to complete. They must also have creativity. The ability to work well as part of a team is also important.

Almost all pharmacologists have a Ph.D. earned from an accredited medical school or school of pharmacy. A bachelor's degree is necessary to be accepted into a graduate program in pharmacology. As undergraduates, students should emphasize the sciences—courses in physical chemistry, biology, organic chemistry, and mathematics are important. Also, courses in English are helpful for preparing students to write research reports.

Completion of a Ph.D. program takes four to six years. Course work will include biomedical sciences, research techniques, and the successful completion of an original research project as well as a doctoral thesis written about the project.

Potential and Advancement

Opportunities for pharmacologists should be very good through the year 2000 due to a general growth in health care and health care-related industries and the demand for pharmacologists to evaluate continually the toxicity or value of various chemicals, drugs, and substances.

Most pharmacologists begin laboratory work in junior positions, working under the supervision of a more experienced pharmacologist. Advancement usually means a supervisory position or managing a major research project. Some pharmacologists become teachers.

Income

Beginning pharmacologists with a Ph.D. have starting salaries that range from $30,000 to $45,000 a year. More experienced workers earn $50,000 or more, and those with an M.D. degree can earn more than $100,000 a year.

Physical Therapist

Additional Sources of Information

American Chemical Society
Career Services
1155 16th Street, NW
Washington, DC 20036

American College of Clinical Pharmacology
175 Strafford Avenue
Suite 1
Wayne, PA 19087

American Society for Pharmacology and Experimental Therapeutics
9650 Rockville Pike
Bethesda, MD 20814

Physical Therapist

The Job At some point in their treatment, accident and stroke victims, handicapped children, and disabled older persons are usually referred by their doctor to a physical therapist. The therapist will design and carry out a program of testing, exercise, massage, or other therapeutic treatment that will increase strength, restore the range of motion, relieve pain, and improve the condition of muscles and skin.

Physical therapists provide direct patient care and usually do their own evaluation of the patient's needs. The physical therapist works, however, in close cooperation with the physician and any other specialists involved in the care of the patient such as vocational therapists, psychologists, and social workers. In large hospitals and nursing homes, physical therapists may carry out a program designed by the director or assistant director of the physical therapy department rather than develop the program themselves. Some physical therapists specialize in one variety of patient such as children or the elderly or one type of condition such as arthritis, amputations, or paralysis.

Most physical therapists work in hospitals. Nursing homes employ a growing number and also use the services of self-employed therapists. Rehabilitation centers, schools for handicapped children, public health agencies, physicians' offices, and the armed forces all employ physical therapists. Some therapists also work with patients in their own homes or provide instructions to the patient and the patient's family on how to continue therapy at home.

Because this field has so many opportunities for part-time practitioners, it appeals to people with family responsibilities.

Places of Employment and Working Conditions

Physical therapists are employed throughout the country, with the largest number working in cities with large hospitals or medical centers.

Since physical therapy, unlike many other medical procedures, does not have to be provided on a 24-hour basis, most therapists work a 40-hour week. In the case of self-employed and part-time therapists, some evening and weekend work may be required.

Qualifications, Education, and Training

Patience, tact, emotional stability, and the ability to work with people are important for anyone interested in this field. Manual dexterity and physical stamina are also important.

High school students considering this field should take courses in health, biology, social science, mathematics, and physical education. Part-time or volunteer work in the physical therapy department of a hospital can provide a closer look at the work for anyone trying to decide on a career in physical therapy.

There are two types of programs for physical therapy training: a four-year bachelor's degree in physical therapy or an entry-level master's degree program.

Physical therapists must be licensed. A degree or certificate from an accredited program and a passing grade on a state board examination completes the requirements for obtaining a license.

Potential and Advancement

There are about 68,000 licensed physical therapists. Employment in the field is expected to expand rapidly as the demand grows for more rehabilitative facilities for accident victims, the elderly, and handicapped children. Opportunities for part-time work will also continue to grow.

As the number of new graduates in the field catches up with the number of job openings, job competition will probably develop in large population centers. Job opportunities will continue to be good in suburban and rural areas, too.

Advancement in this field depends on experience and advanced education especially for teaching, research, and administrative positions.

Income

Newly graduated physical therapists earn about $25,000 a year. Earnings of experienced therapists average about $33,400.

Additional Source of Information

American Physical Therapy Association
1111 North Fairfax Street
Alexandria, VA 22314

Physician

The Job Physicians diagnose diseases, treat illnesses and injuries, and are involved in research, rehabilitation, and preventive medicine.

Most physicians specialize in a particular field of medicine such as internal medicine, general surgery, psychiatry, or pediatrics. The fastest growing specialty is family practice, which emphasizes general medicine.

Most new physicians open their own offices or join associate or group practices. Those who enter the armed forces start with the rank of captain in the army or air force or lieutenant in the navy. Other federal positions are in the Department of Veterans Affairs; the U.S. Public Health Service; and the Department of Health and Human Services.

Places of Employment and Working Conditions

Just about every community has at least one physician.

The northeastern states have the highest ratios of physicians to population; the southern states have the lowest. Physicians tend to locate in urban areas close to hospital facilities and educational centers; rural areas are often underserved.

Many physicians have long and irregular working hours. Specialists work fewer hours than general practitioners. Physicians do have the option of curtailing their practices as they grow older, thus being able to work at a reduced pace past the normal retirement age.

Qualifications, Education, and Training

Anyone interested in this field must have a strong desire to serve the sick and injured. He or she must have emotional stability and the ability to make quick decisions in an emergency and be able to relate well to people. The study of medicine is long and expensive and requires a commitment to intense, vigorous training.

High school should include as much mathematics and science as possible, and grades should average B or above.

Most medical school applicants have a bachelor's degree, although medical schools will accept three years of premedical college study. Competition for entrance into medical school is fierce. Premedical college grades of B or better are usually necessary along with a high grade on the Medical College Admission Test (MCAT). Other relevant factors are the applicant's character, personality, and leadership qualities; letters of recommendation; and, in state-supported medical schools, areas of residence.

It usually takes four years to complete medical school; students with outstanding ability sometimes complete it in three. A few schools have programs that allow completion of premedical and medical studies in a total of six years.

The first half of medical school is spent in classrooms and laboratories studying medical sciences. The remaining time is spent in clinical work under the supervision of experienced physicians. At the completion of medical school, students are awarded a doctor of medicine (M.D.) degree.

After graduation, a three-year hospital residency is usually completed. Those seeking certification in a specialty spend up to five years in advanced residency training; this is followed by two or more years of practice in the specialty before the required specialty board examination is taken.

Physicians who intend to teach or do research must earn a master's or Ph.D. degree in a field such as biochemistry or microbiology.

All physicians must be licensed to practice medicine. Requirements usually include graduation from an accredited medical school, completion of a residency program, and a passing grade on a licensing examination—usually the National Board of Medical Examiners (NBME) test. Applicants who have not taken the NBME test must sit for the Federation Licensing Examination that is accepted by all jurisdictions. Physicians licensed in one state can obtain a license in most other states without further examination.

Graduates of foreign medical schools must pass an examination given by the Educational Commission for Foreign Medical Graduates before they are allowed to serve a residency in the United States.

Potential and Advancement

There are about 535,000 professionally active physicians in the United States. Employment opportunities should be very good through the year 2000 due to the growing demands for health care. Anticipated increases in the number of medical graduates of existing and new U.S. medical schools, combined with foreign medical graduates, could cause the supply to exceed the demand. This should encourage more physicians to establish practices in areas that have traditionally lacked sufficient medical services such as rural and inner-city areas. An increase in the supply of new physicians will also mean more competition in some specialty fields. Primary care practitioners, such as family physicians, pediatricians, and internal medicine specialists, will continue to be in demand.

Physician Assistant

Income Physicians have the highest average annual earnings of any occupational or professional group—about $132,000 a year.

New physicians setting up their own practice usually have a few very lean years in the beginning, but, once a practice is established, earnings rise rapidly. Physicians in a private practice usually earn more than those in salaried positions, and specialists earn considerably more than general practitioners.

Because practitioners in metropolitan areas have much better incomes than those in rural areas, some rural communities offer a guaranteed annual income to a physician who is willing to practice in their area.

Additional Sources of Information

American Medical Association
535 North Dearborn Street
Chicago, IL 60610

Association of American Medical Colleges
Publications Department
One Dupont Circle, NW
Suite 200
Washington, DC 20036

Physician Assistant

The Job Physician assistants, or PAs, relieve primary care physicians of some of their duties. They are trained to perform such medical procedures as taking medical histories, performing physical examinations, making preliminary diagnoses, prescribing treatments, and suggesting medications and drug therapies. In some states, PAs are permitted to prescribe medication.

PAs also treat minor medical problems such as cuts and burns. They provide pre- and postoperative care and sometimes assist in surgery.

PAs work in several medical specialties, including family practice, internal medicine, general and thoracic surgery, emergency medicine, and pediatrics.

Other titles for PAs include MEDEX, surgeon's assistant, child health associate, and physician associate.

Places of Employment and Working Conditions

PAs work in physicians' offices, hospitals, and clinics. Some work in inner-city or rural clinics where a physician comes only once or twice a week. The rest of the week, the PA independently provides health care services after consulting with the supervising physician by telephone.

PAs have varying schedules depending on their work setting. Usually they share the same work hours as their supervising physician. If their employer provides 24-hour medical care, they may be required to work nights, weekends, and holidays.

Qualifications, Education, and Training

PAs should enjoy working with people. Leadership skills, confidence, and emotional stability are also important qualities.

Almost all states require that PAs complete an accredited formal education program. There are currently over 50 educational programs for physician assistants. Most offer a bachelor's degree; others offer a certificate, an associate's degree, or a master's degree.

Admission requirements for many programs include two years of college and work experience in the health field. A number of programs, however, are doing away with requirements for previous work experience.

PA programs are usually two years long. They are offered by medical schools, schools of allied health, and four-year colleges; a few are sponsored by community colleges or hospitals. Course work includes classroom instruction and supervised experience in clinical practice.

Most states have laws concerning the qualifications or practice of PAs and require them to pass a certifying exam given only to graduates of accredited programs.

Potential and Advancement

There are about 48,000 physician assistants. There should be very good opportunities for physician assistants through the year 2000. The health services industry is expected to expand greatly, and PAs will be in demand to relieve doctors of some of their more routine tasks and assist them in more complex medical and surgical procedures.

PAs sometimes advance by taking additional training that allows them to work in a specialty area such as surgery and emergency medicine. Others earn higher salaries and are given more responsibility as they gain experience and increase their knowledge. PAs, though, are always supervised by doctors.

Income

The average starting salary for physician assistants is about $26,500 a year. Experienced physician assistants earn an average salary of about $34,000.

Additional Sources of Information

American Academy of Physician Assistants
950 North Washington Street
Alexandria, VA 22314

American Medical Association
535 North Dearborn Street
Chicago, IL 60610

Podiatrist

The Job The diagnosis and treatment of diseases and deformities of the feet is the special field of podiatrists. They treat corns, bunions, calluses, ingrown toenails, skin and nail diseases, deformed toes, and arch disabilities. If a person's feet show symptoms of medical disorders that affect other parts of the body (such as arthritis or diabetes), the podiatrist will refer the patient to a medical doctor while continuing to treat the patient's foot problem.

In the course of diagnosis, podiatrists may take x-rays and perform blood tests or other pathological tests. They perform surgery; fit corrective devices; and prescribe drugs, physical therapy, and proper shoes.

Most podiatrists provide all types of foot care, but some specialize in foot surgery, orthopedics (bone, muscle, and joint disorders), children's foot ailments, or foot problems of the elderly.

Some podiatrists purchase established practices or spend their early years in a salaried position while gaining experience and earning the money to set up their own practices. Podiatrists in full-time salaried positions usually work in hospitals, podiatric medical colleges, or for other podiatrists. Public health departments and the Department of Veterans Affairs also employ both full- and part-time podiatrists, and some serve as commissioned officers in the armed forces.

Places of Employment and Working Conditions Podiatrists work in all sections of the country but are usually found in or near one of the seven states that have colleges of podiatric medicine.

Most podiatrists are in private practice, work about 40 hours a week, and set their own schedules. They also spend some hours handling the administration and paperwork of their practice. Podiatrists who work for hospitals or HMOs may be required to work nights or weekends. This is not physically strenuous work, a fact that allows practitioners in private practice to work past normal retirement age.

Qualifications, Education, and Training

Anyone interested in a career as a podiatrist should have scientific aptitude, manual dexterity, and an ability to work with people.

High school courses in mathematics and science are important preparation.

The degree of doctor of podiatric medicine (D.P.M.) is available after successful completion of at least three years of college and four years of a school of podiatric medicine. Competition for entry in these schools is strong and, although three years of college is the minimum requirement, most successful applicants have a bachelor's degree and an overall grade point average of B or better. College study must include courses in English, chemistry, biology or zoology, physics, and mathematics. All schools of podiatric medicine also require applicants to take the Medical College Admission Test (MCAT).

The first two years in podiatry school are spent in classroom and laboratory study of anatomy, bacteriology, chemistry, pathology, physiology, pharmacology, and other basic sciences. In the final two years, students obtain clinical experience. Additional study and experience are necessary for practice in a specialty.

All podiatrists must be licensed. Requirements include graduation from an accredited college of podiatric medicine and passing grades on written and oral state board proficiency examinations. Many states also require a residency in a hospital or clinic. A majority of states grant licenses without examination to podiatrists licensed by another state.

Potential and Advancement

There are about 17,000 practicing podiatrists, most of them located in large cities. Employment in this field is expected to grow, and opportunities for graduates to establish new practices or enter salaried positions should be good through the year 2000.

Increasing population, especially the growing number of older people who need foot care and who are covered by Medicare, will contribute to the demand for podiatrists.

Income

Most newly licensed podiatrists set up their own practices and, as in most new practices, earn a great deal less in the early years than they will after a few years in practice. The average yearly income of all podiatrists is about $90,000.

Prosthetist and Orthotist

Additional Sources of Information

American Association of Colleges of Podiatric Medicine
6110 Executive Boulevard
Suite 204
Rockville, MD 20852

American Podiatric Medical Association
6110 Executive Boulevard
Suite 204
Rockville, MD 20852

Prosthetist and Orthotist

The Job Prosthetists work with patients who have lost limbs or partial limbs, and orthotists help patients who have disabled limbs or spines. Prosthetists construct replacement limbs, called prostheses. Orthotists design corrective devices, such as braces, called orthoses.

Prosthetists or orthotists receive a prescription from a physician for patients who have lost a limb or have a handicap. The prosthetist or orthotist then examines the patient and takes the necessary measurements to make sure that the device will fit properly. Each device is designed and constructed to meet a patient's individual needs.

The prosthetists and orthotists then make the device, using power and hand tools and leather, wood, or plastic. Once the device is completed, the prosthetist or orthotist fits it to the patient and makes any necessary adjustments or alterations. He or she then works with other members of the health care team, such as the physician or therapist, to help the patient adjust to the device.

Places of Employment and Working Conditions Prosthetists and orthotists work in departments of prosthetics and orthotics in hospitals, clinics, and rehabilitation centers. Others have their own private practice.

Prosthetists and orthotists usually work in clean, well-lighted offices, examination rooms, and fitting rooms. Lab workers may sometimes have to cope with noise and fumes. Forty-hour, five-day workweeks are typical, with very little overtime work.

Qualifications, Education, and Training

Important qualities for workers in this field include patience, compassion, and creativity. Prosthetists and orthotists should have an aptitude for science and engineering.

A bachelor's degree in prosthetics or orthotics is necessary for work in this field. Course work includes biology, anatomy, physics, and engineering. There is a great deal of lab work, making and fitting devices.

While certification is not required, those who are certified have better opportunities available. The American Board for Certification in Orthotics and Prosthetics certifies those who have a bachelor's degree in prosthetics or orthotics from a board-approved college or university, at least one year of clinical experience, and a passing grade on an exam. Those who meet these qualifications are a certified prosthetist (C.P.), certified orthotist (C.O.), or certified prosthetist-orthotist (C.P.O.).

Potential and Advancement

Because of the growth of the elderly population, better access to medical and rehabilitation care brought about by expanding insurance coverage, and continuing advancement in this field, job opportunities should be good through the year 2000.

Prosthetists and orthotists may advance by becoming heads of departments. Others advance by starting their own private practice. Some become teachers or researchers.

Income

The average starting salary for prosthetists and orthotists is more than $19,000 a year. Those with experience earn between $24,000 and $29,000 a year. Practitioners with certification can earn even more; in hospitals salaries for certified workers range from $30,000 to $36,000.

Additional Sources of Information

American Academy of Orthotists and Prosthetists
717 Pendleton Street
Alexandria, VA 22314

American Board for Certification in Orthotics and Prosthetics
717 Pendleton Street
Alexandria, VA 22314

International Society for Prosthetics and Orthotics
U.S. National Member Society
317 East 34th Street
New York, NY 10016

Psychiatrist

The Job A psychiatrist is a medical doctor (physician) who specializes in the problems of mental illness. Because a psychiatrist is also a physician, he or she is licensed to use a wider variety of treatments—including drugs, hospitalization, somatic (shock) therapy—than others who provide treatment for the mentally ill.

Psychiatrists may specialize as to psychiatric technique and age or type of patients treated.

Most psychiatrists are *psychotherapists* who treat individual patients directly. They sometimes treat patients in groups or in a family group.

This is a technique of verbal therapy and may be supplemented with other treatments such as medication. Some psychiatrists are *psychoanalysts* who specialize in a technique of individual therapy based on the work of Sigmund Freud. Psychiatrists who practice this specialty must themselves undergo psychoanalysis in the course of their training. *Child psychiatrists* specialize in the treatment of children.

Some psychiatrists work exclusively in research, studying such things as the effect of drugs on the brain, or in the basic sciences of human behavior. Others teach at the college and university level. Research and teaching psychiatrists, however, usually combine their work with a certain amount of direct patient care.

In addition to private practice, psychiatrists work in clinics, general hospitals, and private and public psychiatric hospitals. The federal government employs a number of psychiatrists in the Veterans Administration and the U.S. Public Health Service.

Related jobs are psychologist and rehabilitation counselor.

Places of Employment and Working Conditions Psychiatrists work in all parts of the country, almost always in large metropolitan areas or near universities and medical schools.

This field can be emotionally wearing on the psychiatrist. The shortage of psychiatrists and the increasing demand for psychiatric services means that many practitioners are overworked and often cannot devote as much time as they would like to each individual patient.

The expense and time involved in securing an education for this field deters some people from pursuing psychiatry as a career.

Qualifications, Education, and Training More than in any other field, the personality of the psychiatrist is very important. Emotional stability, patience, the ability to empathize with the patient, and a manner that encourages trust and confidence are absolutely necessary. The psychiatrist must be inquisitive, analytical, and flexible in the treatment of patients and must have great self-awareness of his or her own limitations and biases.

A high school student interested in this field should take a college preparatory course strong in science.

After high school, the training of a psychiatrist takes from 12 to 14 years. (Educational requirements for a physician are detailed under that job description.)

After receiving an M.D. degree and completing a one-year medical internship in a hospital approved by the American Medical Association (AMA), a prospective psychiatrist begins a three- to four-year psychiatric specialty program. This program must take place in a hospital approved for this purpose by both the AMA and the American Psychiatric Association.

Training is carried on during a residency program that requires study, research, and clinical practice under the supervision of staff psychiatrists. After completion of the program and two years of experience, a psychiatrist is eligible to take the psychiatry examination of the American Board of Neurology and Psychiatry. Successful applicants then receive a diploma from this specialty board and are considered to be fully qualified psychiatrists.

At this point, a psychiatrist who wishes to specialize in child psychiatry must complete an additional two years of training, usually in a children's psychiatric hospital or clinic. A diploma in child psychiatry is then awarded after successful completion of the required examination.

Psychiatrists must also fulfill state licensing requirements before starting the residency period. Licensing requirements are explained in the job description for physician.

Potential and Advancement

Job opportunities are excellent for psychiatrists through the year 2000. Although there is currently an oversupply in some areas of the United States, some predict a shortage, especially in areas such as child psychiatry.

Psychiatrists may advance by building their practices. Some become experts in a certain field of psychiatry. Those employed in psychiatric hospitals may advance to administrative positions, and those who teach in colleges and universities may advance through the academic ranks to become full professors.

Income

During training, psychiatric residents receive a salary and are often provided with living quarters; their average annual earnings are about $22,000.

Experienced psychiatrists' earnings are similar to other physicians' earnings. Their average yearly salary is about $85,000, with some who work in private practice earning about $200,000 or more a year.

Additional Sources of Information

American Medical Association
535 North Dearborn Street
Chicago, IL 60610

American Psychiatric Association
1400 K Street, NW
Washington, DC 20005

Psychologist

The Job Psychologists study the behavior of individuals and groups to understand and explain their actions. Psychologists gather information through interviews and tests, by studying personal histories, and conducting controlled experiments.

Psychologists may specialize in a wide variety of areas. *Experimental psychologists* study behavior processes by working with human beings as well as rats, monkeys, and pigeons. Their research includes motivation, learning and retention, sensory and perceptual processes, and genetic and neurological factors in human behavior. *Developmental psychologists* study the patterns and causes of behavior change in different age groups. *Personality psychologists* study human nature, individual differences, and the ways in which these differences develop.

Social psychologists examine people's interactions with others and with the social environment. Their studies include group behavior, leadership, and dependency relationships. *Environmental psychologists* study the influence of environments on people; *physiological psychologists* study the relationship of behavior to the biological functions of the body.

Psychologists often combine several of these or other specialty areas in their work. They further specialize in the setting in which they apply their knowledge.

Clinical psychologists work in mental hospitals or clinics or maintain their own practices. They provide individual, family, and group psychotherapy programs. *Counseling psychologists* help people with the problems of daily life—personal, social, educational, or vocational. *Educational psychologists* apply their expertise to problems in education while *school psychologists* work with students and diagnose educational problems, help in adjustment to school, and solve learning and social problems.

Others work as *industrial and organizational psychologists* (personnel work), *engineering psychologists* (human-machine systems), and *consumer psychologists* (what motivates consumers).

About 19,000 psychologists work in colleges and universities as teachers, researchers, administrators, or counselors. Most of the rest work in hospitals, clinics, rehabilitation centers, and other health facilities. The remainder work for federal, state, and local government agencies; correctional institutions; research firms; or in private practice.

Related jobs are psychiatrist, rehabilitation counselor, guidance counselor, marriage counselor, and social worker.

Places of Employment and Working Conditions

Psychologists work in communities of all sizes. The largest concentrations are in areas with colleges and universities.

Working hours for psychologists are flexible in general. Their specialties, however, determine their schedules. Clinical and counseling psychologists, for example, often work in the evening to accommodate the work and school schedules of their patients.

Qualifications, Education, and Training

Sensitivity to others and an interest in people are very important as are emotional stability, patience, and tact. Research requires an interest in detail, accuracy, and communication skills.

High school preparation should emphasize science and social science skills.

A bachelor's degree in psychology or a related field such as social work or education is only a first step, because a Ph.D. is the minimum requirement for employment as a psychologist. Those with only a bachelor's degree will be limited to jobs as research or administrative assistants in mental health centers, vocational rehabilitation offices and correctional programs, government, or business. Some may work as secondary school teachers if they complete state certification requirements.

Stiff competition for admission into graduate psychology programs means that only the most highly qualified applicants are accepted. College grades of B or higher are necessary.

At least one year of graduate study is necessary to earn a master's degree in psychology. Those with a master's degree qualify to work under the supervision of a psychologist and collect and analyze data and administer and interpret some kinds of psychological tests. They may also qualify for certain counseling positions such as school psychologist.

Three to five years of additional graduate work are required to earn a Ph.D. in psychology. Clinical and counseling psychologists need still another year or more of internship or other supervised experience. Some programs also require competence in a foreign language.

A dissertation based on original research that contributes to psychological knowledge is required of Ph.D. candidates. Another degree in this field is the Psy.D. (doctor of psychology). Acquisition of this degree is based on practical work and examinations rather than a dissertation.

The American Board of Professional Psychology awards diplomas in clinical, clinical neuropsychology, counseling, forensic, industrial and organizational, and school psychology. Candidates must have a Ph.D. or Psy.D. and five years of experience, pass an examination, and provide professional endorsements.

State licensing and certification requirements vary but usually require a Ph.D. or Psy.D., one to two years of professional experience, and a written examination.

Potential and Advancement There are about 104,000 people working as psychologists. Employment in this field is expected to grow, but opportunities will be best for those with doctoral degrees.

Traditional academic specialties such as experimental, physiological, and comparative psychology will provide fewer job opportunities than the applied areas of school, clinical, counseling, health, industrial, and engineering psychology.

Income Median salaries for experienced psychologists with doctoral degrees are $42,100 in educational institutions; $40,000 in state and local governments and hospitals and clinics; $34,500 in nonprofit organizations; and $60,100 in business and industry.

Additional Source of Information

American Psychological Association
Educational Affairs Office
1200 17th Street, NW
Washington, DC 20036

Radiologic (X-Ray) Technologist

The Job In the medical field, x-ray pictures (radiographs) are taken by radiologic technologists who operate x-ray equipment. They usually work under the supervision of a radiologist—a physician who specializes in the use and interpretation of x-rays.

There are three specialties within the field of radiologic technology; a radiologic technologist works in all three areas.

The most familiar specialty is the use of x-ray pictures to study and diagnose injury or disease to the human body. In this specialty, the technologist positions the patient and exposes and develops the film. During fluoroscopic examinations (watching the internal movements of the body organs on a screen or monitor), the technologist prepares solutions and assists the physician.

The second specialty area is nuclear medicine technology—the application of radioactive material to aid in the diagnosis and treatment of illness or injury. Working under the direct supervision of a radiologist, the technologist prepares solutions containing radioactive materials that will be absorbed by the patient's internal organs and show up on special cameras or scanners. These materials trace the course of a disease by showing the difference between healthy and diseased tissue.

Radiation therapy—the use of radiation-producing machines to provide therapeutic treatments—is the third specialty. Here, the technologist works under the direct supervision of a radiologist, applying the prescribed amount of radiation for a specified length of time.

During all these procedures, the technologist is responsible for the safety and comfort of the patient and must keep accurate and complete records of all treatments. Technologists also schedule appointments and file x-rays and the radiologist's evaluations.

About three-fifths of all radiological technologists work in hospitals. The remainder work in medical laboratories, physicians' and dentists' offices, federal and state health agencies, and public school systems.

Places of Employment and Working Conditions Radiologic technologists are found in all parts of the country in towns and cities of all sizes. The largest concentrations are in cities with large medical centers and hospitals.

Full-time technologists usually work a 40-hour week. Those employed in hospitals that provide 24-hour emergency coverage have some shift work or may be

Radiologic (X-Ray) Technologist

on call. There are potential radiation hazards in this field, but careful attention to safety procedures and the use of protective clothing and shielding devices provide protection.

Qualifications, Education, and Training Anyone considering this career should be in good health, emotionally stable, and able to work with people who are injured or ill. The job also requires patience and attention to detail.

A high school diploma or its equivalent is required for acceptance into an x-ray technology program. Programs approved by the Committee on Allied Health Education and Accreditation are offered by many hospitals, medical schools affiliated with hospitals, colleges and universities, vocational and technical schools, and the armed forces. The programs vary in length from one to four years; a bachelor's degree in radiologic technology is awarded after completion of the four-year course.

These training programs include courses in anatomy, physiology, patient care procedures, physics, radiation protection, film processing, medical terminology and ethics, radiographic positioning and exposure, and department administration.

Although registration with the American Registry of Radiologic Technologists is not required for work in this field, it is an asset in obtaining highly skilled and specialized positions. Twenty-five states require radiologic technologists to be licensed.

Potential and Advancement There are about 132,000 radiological technologists at the present time. Employment in this field, as in all medical fields, is expected to expand rapidly because of the importance of this technology to diagnosing and treating disease.

In large x-ray departments, technologists can advance to supervisory positions or qualify as instructors in x-ray techniques. There is more opportunity for promotion for those having a bachelor's degree.

Income Starting salaries in hospitals and medical centers average about $18,408 a year. Experienced technologists average about $24,552.

Sick leave, vacation, insurance, and other benefits are usually the same as other employees in the same institution receive.

Additional Source of Information

American Society of Radiologic Technologists
15000 Central Avenue, SE
Albuquerque, NM 87123

Recreational Therapist

The Job Recreational therapy, a fairly new field, uses activities to improve the physical, mental, and emotional health of disabled people. By using activities such as athletic events, dances, arts and crafts, and music, recreational therapists help their patients improve their physical condition, their confidence, their stress management capabilities, and their emotional status. The specific aspects of recreational therapists' jobs, however, depend on their work setting and the type of patients with whom they work.

By talking with patients, their relatives, and other staff members involved in patients' treatment, therapists gather information that will help them determine the best course of treatment for individual patients. Therapists then select a therapeutic activity that complements that patient's interests and enthusiasms.

During the patient's involvement in activities, the therapist closely observes and notes changes and improvements in the patient's condition. The therapist reviews the activity program and determines whether any modifications are necessary as the patient's condition changes or improves. An important part of the therapist's job is recordkeeping—notes on the patient's progress, changes in the treatment plan, staff notes, and discharge notes.

Recreational therapists who work in hospitals provide a more active type of treatment. Those working in other settings, such as nursing homes and community centers, tend to emphasize leisure activities more in assisting their patients.

Recreational therapists are also called therapeutic recreation specialists and, in nursing homes, activities directors.

Places of Employment and Working Conditions

Over one-third of all recreational therapists work in hospitals and nursing homes. Therapists also work in community mental health centers, adult day care programs, correctional facilities, homes for the mentally retarded, community programs, and substance abuse centers. A few therapists are self-employed and oversee programs in nursing homes or community programs on a contract basis.

Recreational Therapist

Working conditions depend on the work setting, facilities, and type of therapy program. Some therapists work in a specially equipped room while others work in a different setting daily or weekly. Therapists usually work a 40-hour week. Working with patients with special needs can be demanding and physically tiring as well if the therapist participates in activities and must lift and carry equipment.

Qualifications, Education, and Training   A desire to help disabled people and patience are important qualities for recreational therapists. Also important are creativity and imagination for determining activities that will meet individual needs.

At this time, hiring requirements vary. For clinical positions, such as those in hospitals, mental health settings, and rehabilitation facilities, a degree in therapeutic recreation is usually required. There are over 200 programs in recreational therapy, and around 60 are accredited by the National Council on Accreditation. Most of these are bachelor's degree programs, but some offer associate's or master's degrees. Course work in these programs includes management, professional issues, human anatomy and physiology, abnormal psychology, and characteristics of illnesses and disabilities.

In nursing homes, often an associate's degree or work experience will qualify an individual for the position of activities director.

A few states monitor this occupation by licensure, certification, or regulation of titles. Typical requirements for licensure include a degree in an accredited therapeutic recreation program, a supervised internship, and passing a state licensing exam.

Potential and Advancement   There are about 26,000 recreational therapists, and opportunities are expected to grow rapidly through the year 2000 due to increased need for long-term care, physical and psychiatric rehabilitation, and services for the mentally and emotionally disabled.

Job growth will also occur in hospitals. Nursing homes, retirement communities, and adult day care will provide many jobs as the number of people age 75 and older increases. Community programs are expected to grow as well.

To advance, recreational therapists need a master's degree. They may become overseers of programs in larger institutions, teachers, or researchers.

Income   Several factors affect salaries: employment setting, educational background, experience, and region. The median annual salary for full-time recreational therapists is $23,500. Average salaries for activities directors in nursing homes range from $15,000 to $25,000 annually. The median annual salary for hospital-employed therapists is about $20,300; experienced therapists earn about $27,600.

Additional Sources of Information

American Therapeutic Recreation Association
C.O. Associated Management Systems
P.O. Box 15215
Hattiesburg, MS 39403

National Council for Therapeutic Recreation Certification
49 South Main Street
Suite 005
Spring Valley, NY 10977

National Therapeutic Recreation Society
3101 Park Center Drive
Alexandria, VA 22302

Rehabilitation Counselor

The Job Rehabilitation counselors work with mentally, physically, and emotionally disabled persons to help them become self-sufficient and productive. Many counselors specialize in one type of disability, such as the mentally retarded, the mentally ill, or the blind.

In the course of designing an individual rehabilitation program, the counselor may consult doctors, teachers, and family members to determine the client's abilities and the exact nature of the handicap or disability. He or she will, of course, also work closely with the client. Many counselors discuss training and career options with the client, arrange specialized training and specific job-related training, and provide encouragement and emotional support.

An important part of a counselor's work is finding employers who will hire the disabled and the handicapped. Many counselors keep in touch with members of the local business community and try to convince them to provide jobs for the disabled. Once a person is placed in a job, the rehabilitation counselor keeps track of the daily progress of the employee and also confers with the employer about job performance and progress.

Rehabilitation Counselor

The amount of time spent with an individual client depends on the severity of the person's problems and the size of the counselor's case load. Counselors in private organizations can usually spend more time with their clients than those who work for state and local agencies. Less-experienced counselors and counselors who work with the severely disabled usually handle the fewest cases at one time.

Most rehabilitation counselors are employed by state or local rehabilitation agencies. Others work in hospitals or sheltered workshops or are employed by insurance companies and labor unions. The Department of Veterans Affairs employs psychologists who act as rehabilitation counselors.

Related jobs are employment counselor, psychologist, and social worker.

Places of Employment and Working Conditions

Rehabilitation counselors work throughout the country with the largest concentrations in metropolitan areas.

A 40-hour workweek is usual, but attendance at community meetings sometimes requires extra hours. A counselor's working hours are not all spent in the office but include trips to prospective employers, training agencies, and clients' homes.

The work of a counselor can be emotionally exhausting and sometimes discouraging.

Qualifications, Education, and Training

Anyone considering this field should have emotional stability, the ability to accept responsibility and work independently, and the ability to motivate and guide other people. Patience is also a necessary characteristic of a rehabilitation counselor because progress often comes slowly over a long period of time.

High school courses in the social sciences should be a part of a college preparatory course.

A bachelor's degree with a major in education, psychology, guidance, or sociology is the minimum requirement. This is sufficient for only a few entry-level jobs.

Advanced degrees in psychology, vocational counseling, or rehabilitation counseling are necessary for almost all jobs in this field.

Most rehabilitation counselors work for state and local government agencies and are required to pass the appropriate civil service examinations before appointment to a position. Many private organizations require counselors to be certified; this is achieved by passing the examinations administered by the Commission on Rehabilitation Counselor Certification.

Potential and Advancement Employment opportunities are expected to be very good, but, since most job openings are in state and local agencies, the employment picture will depend to a great extent on government funding for such services.

Experienced rehabilitation counselors can advance to supervisory and administrative jobs.

Income Beginning salaries range from $350 to $500 a week. Rehabilitation counselors at the highest level of experience earn nearly twice that amount.

Additional Sources of Information

American Rehabilitation Counseling Association
5999 Stevenson Avenue
Alexandria, VA 22304

National Rehabilitation Counseling Association
633 South Washington Street
Alexandria, VA 22314

Respiratory Therapist

The Job Respiratory therapists provide treatment for patients with cardiorespiratory problems. Their role is important and the responsibilities are great.

Respiratory therapists' work includes giving relief to chronic asthma and emphysema sufferers; emergency care in case of heart failure, stroke, drowning, and shock; and treatment of acute respiratory symptoms in cases of head injuries, poisoning, and drug abuse. They must respond swiftly and start treatment quickly because brain damage may occur if a patient stops breathing for three to five minutes, and lack of oxygen for more than nine minutes almost invariably results in death.

In addition to respiratory therapists, the field includes *respiratory technicians* and *respiratory assistants*.

Therapists and technicians perform essentially the same duties, with therapists having greater responsibility for supervision and instruction.

Assistants have little contact with the patients; their duties are usually limited to cleaning, sterilizing, and storing the respiratory equipment used by therapists and technicians.

Respiratory therapists and technicians work as part of a health care team following doctors' instructions. They use special equipment and techniques—respirators, positive-pressure breathing machines, and cardio-pulmonary resuscitation (CPR)—to treat patients. They are also responsible for keeping records of material costs and charges to patients and maintaining and making minor repairs to equipment. All respiratory therapy workers are trained to observe strict safety precautions in the use and testing of respiratory equipment to minimize the danger of fire.

Most respiratory therapists, technicians, and assistants work in hospitals in respiratory, anesthesiology, or pulmonary medicine departments. Others work for nursing homes, ambulance services, and oxygen equipment rental companies.

Places of Employment and Working Conditions

Respiratory therapy workers are employed in hospitals throughout the country in communities of all sizes. The largest number of job opportunities exists in large metropolitan areas that support several hospitals or large medical centers.

Respiratory therapy workers usually work a 40-hour week and may be required to work evenings, nights, or weekends. Respiratory therapists spend much of their working time on their feet and experience a great deal of stress. They must be careful when working with gases, and they run the risk of catching an infectious disease.

Qualifications, Education, and Training

Anyone interested in entering this field should enjoy working with people and have a patient and understanding manner. The ability to follow instructions and work as a member of a team is important. Manual dexterity and some mechanical ability are necessary in the operation and maintenance of the sometimes complicated respiratory therapy equipment.

High school students interested in this field should take courses in health, biology, mathematics, physics, and bookkeeping.

Formal training in respiratory therapy is necessary for entering the field. There are about 255 institutions that offer programs approved by the Committee on Allied Health Education and Accreditation (CAHEA). All these programs require a high school diploma. Courses may vary from two to four years and include both classroom and clinical work. Students study anatomy and physiology, chemistry, physics, microbiology, and mathematics. A bachelor's degree is awarded to those completing a four-year program, with an associate's degree awarded from some of the shorter programs.

Some respiratory therapists are *registered respiratory therapists* (RRTs). They obtain this designation by completing an examination of the National Board for Respiratory Care and meeting education and experience requirements.

Respiratory technicians can receive certification as a *certified respiratory technician* (CRTT) if they have completed a CAHEA-approved technical training program and have one year of experience. They must pass a single written examination. All respiratory technicians are certified as CRTTs.

Potential and Advancement There are currently about 56,000 therapists. The field is growing rapidly. Growth of health care services in general and the expanding use of respiratory therapy and equipment by hospitals, ambulance services, and nursing homes make this a good job opportunity area, as more and more respiratory specialists are hired to release nurses and other personnel from respiratory therapy duties.

Advancement in this field depends on experience and additional education. Respiratory assistants can advance to the technician or therapist level by completing the required courses; technicians can advance by achieving certification or completing education and testing requirements for the therapist level.

Respiratory therapists can be promoted to assistant chief or chief therapist. With graduate study they can qualify for teaching positions.

Income Starting salary for respiratory therapists in hospitals and medical centers is about $19,632 a year; experienced therapists earn an average of $25,764 a year.

Additional Sources of Information

American Association for Respiratory Care
11030 Ables Lane
Dallas, TX 75229

The National Board for Respiratory Care, Inc.
11015 West 75th Terrace
Shawnee Mission, KS 66214

Speech Pathologist and Audiologist

The Job Speech pathologists and audiologists evaluate speech and hearing disorders and provide treatment. Speech pathologists work with children and adults who have speech, language, and voice disorders because of hearing loss, brain injury, cleft palate, mental retardation, emotional problems, or foreign dialect. Audiologists assess and treat hearing problems. Speech and audiology are so interrelated that expertise in one field requires thorough knowledge of both.

Almost half of all speech pathologists and audiologists work in public schools; colleges and universities employ large numbers in teaching and research. The remainder work in hospitals, clinics, government agencies, industry, and private practice.

Places of Employment and Working Conditions Speech pathologists and audiologists are employed throughout the country with most of them located in urban areas.

Speech pathologists and audiologists usually work at a desk or table in an office setting. While the job is not physically strenuous, it does require concentration and attention to detail and can be mentally exhausting. Some speech pathologists and audiologists work at several different facilities and spend a lot of time traveling.

Qualifications, Education, and Training Patience is an extremely important characteristic for anyone who wants to work in this field since progress is usually very slow. The therapist must also be able to encourage and motivate the clients who are often frustrated by the inability to speak properly. Objectivity and the ability to take responsibility and work with detail are also necessary.

High school should include a strong science background.

A bachelor's degree with a major in speech and hearing or in a related field such as education or psychology is the usual preparation for graduate work.

Most jobs in this field require a master's degree. Graduate study includes supervised clinical training as well as advanced study.

The American Speech and Hearing Association confers a certificate of clinical competence (CCC) on those who have a master's degree, complete a one-year internship, and pass a written examination. Certification is usually necessary to advance professionally.

In 37 states, speech pathologists and audiologists must be licensed.

Potential and Advancement   There are about 53,000 speech pathologists and audiologists. The field is expected to grow as a result of population growth among those age 75 and older, the trend toward earlier recognition and treatment of hearing and language problems in children, recent laws requiring services for the handicapped, and the expanded coverage of Medicare and Medicaid programs. Any decreases in government-funded programs could change this employment picture.

If present trends continue, the increasing number of degrees being awarded in this field may cause some job competition in large metropolitan areas. Job opportunities will continue to be good in smaller cities and towns.

Those with only a bachelor's degree will find very limited job opportunities; advancement will be possible only for those with graduate degrees.

Income   Starting salaries for speech pathologists and audiologists in hospitals are about $25,000 a year. Experienced speech pathologists in hospitals earn about $33,000, and experienced audiologists earn about $37,000.

Most speech pathologists and audiologists working in schools are classified as teachers and are paid similar salaries.

Additional Source of Information

American Speech-Language-Hearing Association
10801 Rockville Pike
Rockville, MD 20852

Surgical Technologist

The Job   Surgical technologists, also called surgical technicians or operating room technicians, provide general assistance to doctors and nurses before, during, and after a surgical procedure. Before an operation, surgical technologists prepare the operating room by making sure that surgical instruments, equipment, sterile linens, and fluids are in place. They also may get patients

Surgical Technologist

ready for surgery by washing, shaving, and disinfecting areas on which the surgeon will operate. They then transport patients to the operating room, position them on the operating table, and help drape them.

During surgery, they assist surgeons by passing them sterile instruments and other supplies. They may be required to hold retractors, cut sutures, and help count equipment used during the surgery such as sponges and needles. Specimens taken for laboratory analysis must be prepared, cared for, and disposed of—often the surgical technologists may have to operate some of the equipment used during the surgery.

After a surgery, technologists take patients to the recovery room and assist nurses in seeing that the operating room is restocked with the necessary supplies.

Places of Employment and Working Conditions

Most surgical technologists work in hospitals or facilities where there are operating rooms, delivery rooms, or emergency rooms.

Technologists work in a clean, well-lighted, cool environment. The job may be physically and mentally demanding—technologists sometimes must stay on their feet and remain alert and able to concentrate for surgeries that sometimes last several hours.

Technologists usually work 40-hour, five-day weeks. Since emergency surgery is performed around the clock, technologists may have to be on call during weekends and evenings.

Qualifications, Education, and Training

Those interested in being surgical technologists must have good manual dexterity for handling instruments. Technologists must be conscientious, able to concentrate, and able to work well under pressure.

Almost all technologists are trained in formal education programs offered by community and junior colleges, vocational and technical institutes, or hospitals. There are currently around 200 programs, and a little over half are accredited by the Committee on Allied Health Education and Accreditation of the American Medical Association. Most programs last from nine to ten months, but some community college programs last two years; those who complete a two-year program are granted associate's degrees.

Students in these programs receive instruction in anatomy and physiology, microbiology, pharmacology, and medical terminology. Students also learn how to care for patients during surgery; sterilization techniques; and how to handle certain drugs, equipment, solutions, and supplies.

Potential and Advancement There are about 35,000 technologists currently, and this field is expected to grow rapidly through the year 2000. The rate of surgery is expected to climb as a large percentage of the population grows older, technological advances allow for more surgical intervention for numerous conditions, and insurance companies offer more widespread coverage for surgical care.

Many technologists advance by leaving the field altogether and becoming salespeople; consumer relations specialists; or managers for insurance companies, sterile supply services, or operating equipment firms. They may become instructors in surgical technology programs or, with more education, become registered nurses.

Income Average starting salary for surgical technologists is about $14,928 a year, with more experienced workers earning about $20,124. Salaries vary according to geographical location, with workers on the East and West coasts earning more. Technologists employed by surgeons rather than hospitals tend to earn more.

Additional Source of Information

Association of Surgical Technologists
8307 Shaffer Parkway
Littleton, CO 80127

Veterinarian

The Job Doctors of veterinary medicine diagnose, treat, and control diseases and injuries of animals. They treat animals in hospitals and clinics and on farms and ranches. They perform surgery and prescribe and administer drugs and vaccines.

While most familiar to the general public are those veterinarians who treat small animals and pets exclusively, others specialize in the health and breeding of cattle, horses, and other farm animals. Veterinarians are also employed by federal and state public health programs where they function as meat and poul-

Veterinarian

try inspectors. Others teach at veterinary colleges; do research on animal foods, diseases, and drugs; or take part in medical research for the treatment of human diseases. Veterinarians are also employed by zoos, large animal farms, horse racing stables, and drug manufacturers.

In the army, the air force, and the U.S. Public Health Service, veterinarians are commissioned officers. Other federally employed veterinarians work for the Department of Agriculture.

Places of Employment and Working Conditions

Veterinarians are located throughout the country—in rural areas, small towns, cities, and suburban areas.

Working hours are often long and irregular, and those who work primarily with farm animals must work outdoors in all kinds of weather. In the course of their work, all veterinarians are exposed to injury, disease, and infection.

Qualifications, Education, and Training

A veterinarian needs the ability to get along with animals and should have an interest in science. Physical stamina and a certain amount of strength are also necessary.

High school students interested in this field should emphasize science courses, especially biology. Summer jobs that involve the care of animals can provide valuable experience.

The veterinary degree program (D.V.M. or V.M.D.) requires a minimum of six years of college—at least two years of preveterinary study with emphasis on physical and biological sciences followed by a four-year professional degree program. Most successful applicants complete four years of college before entering the professional program.

There are only 27 accredited colleges of veterinary medicine, many of them state supported. Admission to all of these schools is highly competitive with many more qualified applicants than the schools can accept. Successful applicants need preveterinary college grades of B or better, especially in science courses; part-time work or summer job experience working with animals is a plus. State-supported colleges usually give preference to residents of the state and to applicants from nearby states or regional areas.

The course of study in veterinary colleges is rigorous. It consists of classroom work and practical experience in diagnosing and treating animal diseases, surgery, laboratory work in anatomy and biochemistry, and other scientific and medical studies. Veterinarians who intend to teach or do research usually go on to earn a master's degree in pathology, physiology, or bacteriology.

All states and the District of Columbia require veterinarians to be licensed. Licensing requires a doctor of veterinary medicine degree from an accredited college and passing a written state board of proficiency examination. Some states will issue licenses without examination to veterinarians licensed by another state.

Potential and Advancement   There are about 46,000 active veterinarians, most of them in private practice. Employment opportunities for veterinarians are excellent primarily because of growth in the population of companion animals—horses, dogs, and other pets—and an increase in veterinary research. The growing emphasis on scientific methods of breeding and raising livestock and poultry as well as an increase in public health and disease control programs will also contribute to the demand for veterinarians.

Income   The income of veterinarians in private practice varies greatly depending on type of practice, years of experience, and size and location of community. They usually have higher incomes, however, than veterinarians in salaried positions. The average starting salary for veterinarians is $23,000 a year. More experienced veterinarians' salaries range from $40,000 to $60,000 a year.

Additional Source of Information

American Veterinary Medical Association
930 North Meacham Road
Schaumburg, IL 60196

Appendix

Resumes, Application Forms, Cover Letters, and Interviews

You might see a hurdle to leap over, a hoop to jump through, or a barrier to knock down. That is how many people think of resumes, application forms, cover letters, and interviews. But you do not have to think of them that way. They are not ways to keep you from a job; they are ways for you to show an employer what you know and what you can do. After all, you are going to get a job. It is just a question of which one.

Employers want to hire people who can do the job. To learn who these people are, they use resumes, application forms, written tests, performance tests, medical examinations, and interviews. You can use each of these different evaluation procedures to your advantage. You might not be able to make a silk purse out of a sow's ear, but at least you can show what a good ear you have.

Creating Effective Resumes and Application Forms

Resumes and application forms are two ways to achieve the same goal: to give the employer written evidence of your qualifications. When creating a resume or completing an application form, you need two different kinds of information: facts about yourself and facts about the job you want. With this information in hand, you can present the facts about yourself in terms of the job. You have more freedom with a resume—you can put your best points first and avoid

---

This article is reprinted from *Occupational Outlook Quarterly*, spring 1987, volume 31, number 1, pp. 17-23, written by Neale Baxter.

Appendix

blanks. But, even on application forms, you can describe your qualifications in terms of the job's duties.

Know thyself

Begin by assembling information about yourself. Some items appear on virtually every resume or application form, including the following:

- ◊ Current address and phone number—if you are rarely at home during business hours, try to give the phone number of a friend or relative who will take messages for you.
- ◊ Job sought or career goal.
- ◊ Experience (paid and volunteer)—date of employment, name and full address of the employer, job title, starting and finishing salary, and reason for leaving (moving, returning to school, and seeking a better position are among the readily accepted reasons).
- ◊ Education—the school's name, the city in which it is located, the years you attended it, the diploma or certificate you earned, and the course of studies you pursued.
- ◊ Other qualifications—hobbies, organizations you belong to, honors you have received, and leadership positions you have held.
- ◊ Office machines, tools, equipment you have used, and skills that you possess.

Other information, such as your Social Security number, is often asked for on application forms but is rarely presented on resumes. Application forms might also ask for a record of past addresses and for information that you would rather not reveal, such as a record of convictions. If asked for such information, you must be honest. Honesty does not, however, require that you reveal disabilities that do not affect your overall qualifications for a job.

Know thy job

Next, gather specific information about the jobs you are applying for. You need to know the pay range (so you can make their top your bottom), education and experience usually required, hours and shifts usually worked. Most importantly, you need to know the job duties (so that you can describe your experience in terms of those duties). Study the job description. Some job announcements, especially those issued by a government, even have a checklist that assigns a numerical weight to different qualifications so that you can be certain as to which is the most important; looking at such announcements will give you an idea of what employers look for even if you do not wish to apply for a government job. If the announcement or ad is vague, call the employer to learn what is sought.

Once you have the information you need, you can prepare a resume. You may need to prepare more than one master resume if you are going to look for different kinds of jobs. Otherwise, your resume will not fit the job you seek.

Two kinds of resumes

The way you arrange your resume depends on how well your experience seems to prepare you for the position you want. Basically, you can either describe your most recent job first and work backwards (reverse chronology) or group similar skills together. No matter which format you use, the following advice applies generally.

- ◇ Use specifics. A vague description of your duties will make only a vague impression.
- ◇ Identify accomplishments. If you headed a project, improved productivity, reduced costs, increased membership, or achieved some other goal, say so.
- ◇ Type your resume, using a standard typeface. (Printed resumes are becoming more common, but employers do not indicate a preference for them.)
- ◇ Keep the length down to two pages at the most.
- ◇ Remember your mother's advice not to say anything if you cannot say something nice. Leave all embarrassing or negative information off the resume—but be ready to deal with it in a positive fashion at the interview.
- ◇ Proofread the master copy carefully.
- ◇ Have someone else proofread the master copy carefully.
- ◇ Have a third person proofread the master copy carefully.
- ◇ Use the best quality photocopying machine and good white or off-white paper.

The following information appears on almost every resume.

- ◇ Name.
- ◇ Phone number at which you can be reached or receive messages.
- ◇ Address.
- ◇ Job or career sought.

Appendix

- ◇ References—often just a statement that references are available suffices. If your references are likely to be known by the person who reads the resume, however, their names are worth listing.
- ◇ Experience.
- ◇ Education.
- ◇ Special talents.
- ◇ Personal information—height, weight, marital status, physical condition. Although this information appears on virtually every sample resume I have ever seen, it is not important according to recruiters. In fact, employers are prohibited by law from asking for some of it. If some of this information is directly job related—the height and weight of a bouncer is important to a disco owner, for example—list it. Otherwise, save space and put in more information about your skills.

Reverse chronology is the easiest method to use. It is also the least effective because it makes when you did something more important than what you can do. It is an especially poor format if you have gaps in your work history, if the job you seek is very different from the job you currently hold, or if you are just entering the job market. About the only time you would want to use such a resume is when you have progressed up a clearly defined career ladder and want to move up a rung.

Resumes that are not chronological may be called functional, analytical, skill oriented, creative, or some other name. The differences are less important than the similarity, which is that all stress what you can do. The advantage to a potential employer—and, therefore, to your job campaign—should be obvious. The employer can see immediately how you will fit the job. This format also has advantages for many job hunters because it camouflages gaps in paid employment and avoids giving prominence to irrelevant jobs.

You begin writing a functional resume by determining the skills the employer is looking for. Again, study the job description for this information. Next, review your experience and education to see when you demonstrated the ability sought. Then prepare the resume itself, putting first the information that relates most obviously to the job. The result will be a resume with headings such as "Engineering," "Computer Languages," "Communications Skills," or "Design Experience." These headings will have much more impact than the dates that you would use on a chronological resume.

Fit yourself to a form

Some large employers, such as fast food restaurants and government agencies, make more use of application forms than of resumes. The forms suit the style of large organizations because people find information more quickly if it always appears in the same place. However, creating a resume before filling out an application form will still benefit you. You can use the resume when you send a letter inquiring about a position. You can submit a resume even if an application is required; it will spotlight your qualifications. And the information on the resume will serve as a handy reference if you must fill out an application form quickly. Application forms are really just resumes in disguise anyway. No matter how rigid the form appears to be, you can still use it to show why you are the person for the job being filled.

At first glance, application forms seem to give a job hunter no leeway. The forms certainly do not have the flexibility that a resume does, but you can still use them to your best advantage. Remember that the attitude of the person reading the form is not, "Let's find out why this person is unqualified," but, "Maybe this is the person we want." Use all the parts of the form—experience blocks, education blocks, and others—to show that that person is you.

Here's some general advice on completing application forms.

- ◇ Request two copies of the form. If only one is provided, photocopy it before you make a mark on it. You'll need more than one copy to prepare rough drafts.

- ◇ Read the whole form before you start completing it.

- ◇ Prepare a master copy if the same form is used by several divisions within the same company or organization. Do not put the specific job applied for, date, and signature on the master copy. Fill in that information on the photocopies as you submit them.

- ◇ Type the form if possible. If it has lots of little lines that are hard to type within, type the information on a piece of blank paper that will fit in the space, paste the paper over the form, and photocopy the finished product. Such a procedure results in a much neater, easier to read page.

- ◇ Leave no blanks; enter n/a (for "not applicable") when the information requested does not apply to you; this tells people checking the form that you did not simply skip the question.

- ◇ Carry a resume and a copy of other frequently asked information (such as previous addresses) with you when visiting potential employers in case you must fill out an application on the spot. Whenever possible, however, fill the form out at home and mail it in with a resume and a cover letter that point up your strengths.

Writing Intriguing Cover Letters

You will need a cover letter whenever you send a resume or application form to a potential employer. The letter should capture the employer's attention, show

Appendix

why you are writing, indicate why your employment will benefit the company, and ask for an interview. The kind of specific information that must be included in a letter means that each must be written individually. Each letter must also be typed perfectly, which may present a problem. Word processing equipment helps. Frequently only the address, first paragraph, and specifics concerning an interview will vary. These items are easily changed on word processing equipment and memory typewriters. If you do not have access to such equipment, you might be able to rent it. Or you might be able to have your letters typed by a resume or employment services company listed in the yellow pages. Be sure you know the full cost of such a service before agreeing to use one.

Let's go through a letter point by point.

Salutation

Each letter should be addressed by name to the person you want to talk with. That person is the one who can hire you. This is almost certainly not someone in the personnel department, and it is probably not a department head either. It is most likely to be the person who will actually supervise you once you start work. Call the company to make sure you have the right name. And spell it correctly.

Opening

The opening should appeal to the reader. Cover letters are sales letters. Sales are made after you capture a person's attention. You capture the reader's attention most easily by talking about the company rather than yourself. Mention projects under development, recent awards, or favorable comments recently published about the company. You can find such information in the business press, including the business section of local newspapers and the many magazines that are devoted to particular industries. If you are answering an ad, you may mention it. If someone suggested that you write, use their name (with permission, of course).

Body

The body of the letter gives a brief description of your qualifications and refers to the resume, where your sales campaign can continue.

Closing

You cannot have what you do not ask for. At the end of the letter, request an interview. Suggest a time and state that you will confirm the appointment. Use a standard complimentary close, such as "Sincerely yours," leave three or four lines for your signature, and type your name. I would type my phone number under my name; this recommendation is not usually made, although phone numbers are found on most letterheads. The alternative is to place the phone number in the body of the letter, but it will be more difficult to find there should the reader wish to call you.

Triumphing on Tests and at Interviews

A man with a violin case stood on a subway platform in The Bronx. He asked a conductor, "How do you get to Carnegie Hall?" The conductor replied, "Practice! Practice! Practice!"

Tests

That old joke holds good advice for people preparing for employment tests or interviews. The tests given to job applicants fall into four categories: general aptitude tests, practical tests, tests of physical agility, and medical examinations. You can practice for the first three. If the fourth is required, learn as soon as possible what the disqualifying conditions are, then have your physician examine you for them so that you do not spend years training for a job that you will not be allowed to hold.

To practice for a test, you must learn what the test is. Once again, you must know what job you want to apply for and for whom you want to work in order to find out what tests, if any, are required. Government agencies, which frequently rely on tests, will often provide a sample of the test they use. These samples can be helpful even if an employer uses a different test. Copies of standard government tests are usually available at the library.

If you practice beforehand, you'll be better prepared and less nervous on the day of the test. That will put you ahead of the competition. You will also improve your performance by following this advice:

◊ Make a list of what you will need at the test center, including a pencil; check it before leaving the house.

◊ Get a good night's sleep.

◊ Be at the test center early—at least 15 minutes early.

◊ Read the instructions carefully; make sure they do not differ from the samples you practiced with.

◊ Generally, speed counts; do not linger over difficult questions.

◊ Learn if guessing is penalized. Most tests are scored by counting up the right answers; guessing is all to the good. Some tests are scored by counting the right answers and deducting partial credit for wrong answers; blind

Appendix

guessing will lose you points—but if you can eliminate two wrong choices, a guess might still pay off.

Interviews

For many of us, interviews are the most fearsome part of finding a job. But they are also our best chance to show an employer our qualifications. Interviews are far more flexible than application forms or tests. Use that flexibility to your advantage. As with tests, you can reduce your anxiety and improve your performance by preparing for your interviews ahead of time.

Begin by considering what interviewers want to know. You represent a risk to the employer. A hiring mistake is expensive in terms of lost productivity, wasted training money, and the cost of finding a replacement. To lessen the risk, interviewers try to select people who are highly motivated, understand what the job entails, and show that their background has prepared them for it.

You show that you are highly motivated by learning about the company before the interview, by dressing appropriately, and by being well mannered—which means that you greet the interviewer by name, you do not chew gum or smoke, you listen attentively, and you thank the interviewer at the end of the session. You also show motivation by expressing interest in the job at the end of the interview.

You show that you understand what the job entails and that you can perform it when you explain how your qualifications prepare you for specific duties as described in the company's job listing and when you ask intelligent questions about the nature of the work and the training provided new workers.

One of the best ways to prepare for an interview is to have some practice sessions with a friend or two. Here is a list of some of the most commonly asked questions to get you started.

◊ Why did you apply for this job?

◊ What do you know about this job or company?

◊ Why should I hire you?

◊ What would you do if... (usually filled in with a work-related crisis)?

◊ How would you describe yourself?

◊ What would you like to tell me about yourself?

◊ What are your major strengths?

◊ What are your major weaknesses?

◊ What type of work do you like to do best?

◊ What are your interests outside work?

Appendix

- ◇ What type of work do you like to do least?
- ◇ What accomplishment gave you the greatest satisfaction?
- ◇ What was your worst mistake?
- ◇ What would you change in your past life?
- ◇ What courses did you like best or least in school?
- ◇ What did you like best or least about your last job?
- ◇ Why did you leave your last job?
- ◇ Why were you fired?
- ◇ How does your education or experience relate to this job?
- ◇ What are your goals?
- ◇ How do you plan to reach them?
- ◇ What do you hope to be doing in 5 years? 10?
- ◇ What salary do you expect?

Many jobhunting books available at libraries discuss ways to answer these questions. Essentially, your strategy should be to concentrate on the job and your ability to do it no matter what the question seems to be asking. If asked for a strength, mention something job related. If asked for a weakness, mention a job-related strength (you work too hard, you worry too much about details, you always have to see the big picture). If asked about a disability or a specific negative factor in your past—a criminal record, a failure in school, being fired—be prepared to stress what you learned from the experience, how you have overcome the shortcoming, and how you are now in a position to do a better job.

So far, only the interviewer's questions have been discussed. But an interview will be a two-way conversation. You really do need to learn more about the position to find out if you want the job. Given how frustrating it is to look for a job, you do not want to take just any position only to learn after 2 weeks that you cannot stand the place and have to look for another job right away. Here are some questions for you to ask the interviewer.

- ◇ What would a day on this job be like?
- ◇ Whom would I report to? May I meet this person?
- ◇ Would I supervise anyone? May I meet them?
- ◇ How important is this job to the company?
- ◇ What training programs are offered?

Appendix

- ◇ What advancement opportunities are offered?
- ◇ Why did the last person leave this job?
- ◇ What is that person doing now?
- ◇ What is the greatest challenge of this position?
- ◇ What plans does the company have with regard to...? (Mention some development of which you have read or heard.)
- ◇ Is the company growing?

After you ask such questions, listen to the interviewer's answers and then, if at all possible, point to something in your education or experience related to it. You might notice that questions about salary and fringe benefits are not included in the above list. Your focus at a first interview should be the company and what you will do for it, not what it will pay you. The salary range will often be given in the ad or position announcement, and information on the usual fringe benefits will be available from the personnel department. Once you have been offered a position, you can negotiate the salary. The jobhunting guides available in bookstores and at the library give many more hints on this subject.

At the end of the interview, you should know what the next step will be: Whether you should contact the interviewer again, whether you should provide more information, whether more interviews must be conducted, and when a final decision will be reached. Try to end on a positive note by reaffirming your interest in the position and pointing out why you will be a good choice to fill it.

Immediately after the interview, make notes of what went well and what you would like to improve. To show your interest in the position, send a followup letter to the interviewer, providing further information on some point raised in the interview and thanking the interviewer once again. Remember, someone is going to hire you; it might be the person you just talked to.

VGM CAREER BOOKS

OPPORTUNITIES IN
Available in both paperback and hardbound editions
Accounting
Acting
Advertising
Aerospace
Agriculture
Airline
Animal and Pet Care
Architecture
Automotive Service
Banking
Beauty Culture
Biological Sciences
Biotechnology
Book Publishing
Broadcasting
Building Construction Trades
Business Communication
Business Management
Cable Television
Carpentry
Chemical Engineering
Chemistry
Child Care
Chiropractic Health Care
Civil Engineering
Cleaning Service
Commercial Art and Graphic Design
Computer Aided Design and Computer Aided Mfg.
Computer Maintenance
Computer Science
Counseling & Development
Crafts
Culinary
Customer Service
Dance
Data Processing
Dental Care
Direct Marketing
Drafting
Electrical Trades
Electronic and Electrical Engineering
Electronics
Energy
Engineering
Engineering Technology
Environmental
Eye Care
Fashion
Fast Food
Federal Government
Film
Financial
Fire Protection Services
Fitness
Food Services
Foreign Language
Forestry
Gerontology
Government Service
Graphic Communications
Health and Medical
High Tech
Home Economics
Hospital Administration
Hotel & Motel Management
Human Resources Management Careers
Information Systems
Insurance
Interior Design
International Business
Journalism
Laser Technology
Law
Law Enforcement and Criminal Justice
Library and Information Science
Machine Trades
Magazine Publishing
Management
Marine & Maritime
Marketing
Materials Science
Mechanical Engineering
Medical Technology
Metalworking
Microelectronics
Military
Modeling
Music
Newspaper Publishing
Nursing
Nutrition
Occupational Therapy
Office Occupations
Opticianry
Optometry
Packaging Science
Paralegal Careers
Paramedical Careers
Part-time & Summer Jobs
Performing Arts
Petroleum
Pharmacy
Photography
Physical Therapy
Physician
Plastics
Plumbing & Pipe Fitting
Podiatric Medicine
Postal Service
Printing
Property Management
Psychiatry
Psychology
Public Health
Public Relations
Purchasing
Real Estate
Recreation and Leisure
Refrigeration and Air Conditioning
Religious Service
Restaurant
Retailing
Robotics
Sales
Sales & Marketing
Secretarial
Securities
Social Science
Social Work
Speech-Language Pathology
Sports & Athletics
Sports Medicine
State and Local Government
Teaching
Technical Communications
Telecommunications
Television and Video
Theatrical Design & Production
Transportation
Travel
Trucking
Veterinary Medicine
Visual Arts
Vocational and Technical
Warehousing
Waste Management
Welding
Word Processing
Writing
Your Own Service Business

CAREERS IN Accounting; Advertising; Business; Communications; Computers; Education; Engineering; Health Care; High Tech; Law; Marketing; Medicine; Science

CAREER DIRECTORIES
Careers Encyclopedia
Dictionary of Occupational Titles
Occupational Outlook Handbook

CAREER PLANNING
Admissions Guide to Selective Business Schools
Career Planning and Development for College Students and Recent Graduates
Careers Checklists
Careers for Animal Lovers
Careers for Bookworms
Careers for Culture Lovers
Careers for Foreign Language Aficionados
Careers for Good Samaritans
Careers for Gourmets
Careers for Nature Lovers
Careers for Numbers Crunchers
Careers for Sports Nuts
Careers for Travel Buffs
Guide to Basic Resume Writing
Handbook of Business and Management Careers
Handbook of Health Care Careers
Handbook of Scientific and Technical Careers
How to Change Your Career
How to Choose the Right Career
How to Get and Keep Your First Job
How to Get into the Right Law School
How to Get People to Do Things Your Way
How to Have a Winning Job Interview
How to Land a Better Job
How to Make the Right Career Moves
How to Market Your College Degree
How to Prepare a *Curriculum Vitae*
How to Prepare for College
How to Run Your Own Home Business
How to Succeed in Collge
How to Succeed in High School
How to Write a Winning Resume
Joyce Lain Kennedy's Career Book
Planning Your Career of Tomorrow
Planning Your College Education
Planning Your Military Career
Planning Your Young Child's Education
Resumes for Advertising Careers
Resumes for College Students & Recent Graduates
Resumes for Communications Careers
Resumes for Education Careers
Resumes for High School Graduates
Resumes for High Tech Careers
Resumes for Sales and Marketing Careers
Successful Interviewing for College Seniors

SURVIVAL GUIDES
Dropping Out or Hanging In
High School Survival Guide
College Survival Guide

VGM Career Horizons
a division of *NTC Publishing Group*
4255 West Touhy Avenue
Lincolnwood, Illinois 60646-1975